Sport Medicine: Physiology

A Volume in MSS' Series on Sport Medicine

Papers by
Kenneth D. Rose, Roy J. Shephard, W. P.
Leary et al.

MSS Information Corporation
655 Madison Avenue, New York, N. Y. 10021

Library of Congress Cataloging in Publication Data
Main entry under title:

Sport medicine.

A collection of articles previously published in
various journals.
1. Sports--Physiological aspects--Addresses, essays,
lectures. 2. Athletes--Hygiene--Addresses, essays,
lectures. I. Rose, Kenneth Dwight, 1912-
[DNLM: 1. Sport medicine--Collected works. QT260
R796s 1973]
RC1235.S65   612'.044   73-11032
ISBN 0-8422-7139-2

TABLE OF CONTENTS

CREDITS AND ACKNOWLEDGEMENTS

Andersen, Harald T., "Cardiovascular Adaptations in Diving Mammals," *American Heart Journal*, 1967, 74:295-298.

Baba, Nobuhisa; and Richard D. Ruppert, "Alteration of Eccrine Sweat Gland in Fatal Heat Stroke: Electron Microscopic Observation," *Archives of Pathology*, 1968, 85:669-674.

Byrne-Quinn, Edward; and Robert F. Grover, "Running toward Olympus," *The Lancet*, 1968, 2:1079.

Goodwin, A.B.; and Gordon R. Cumming, "Radio Telemetry of the Electrocardiogram, Fitness Tests, and Oxygen Uptake of Water-Polo Players," *The Canadian Medical Association Journal*, 1966, 95:402-406.

Hughes, John R.; and D. Eugene Hendrix, "Telemetered EEG from a Football Player in Action," *Electroencephalography and Clinical Neurophysiology*, 1968, 24:183-186.

Irvine, C.H.G., "Effect of Exercise on Thyroxine Degradation in Athletes and Non-Athletes," *Journal of Clinical Endocrinology*, 1968, 28:942-948.

Johnson, J., "The EEG in the Traumatic Encephalopathy of Boxers," *Psychiatric Clinics*, 1969, 2:204-211.

Johnson, R.H.; J.L. Walton; H.A. Krebs; and D.H. Williamson, "Metabolic Fuels during and after Severe Exercise in Athletes and Non-Athletes," *The Lancet*, 1969, 2:452-455.

Kuramoto, Kizuku; Michio Ikai; Kazuo Asahina; Yoshio Kuroda; Shinkichi Ogawa; and Mitsumasa Miyashita, "Strenuous Exercise Electrocardiogram of Top Class Swimmers in Mexico City," *Japanese Heart Journal*, 1967, 8:291-300.

Leary, W.P.; and C.H. Wyndham, "The Possible Effect on Athletic Performances of Mexico City's Altitude," *South African Medical Journal*, 1966, 40:984-985.

Leary, W.P.; and J.L. McKechnie, "The Electrocardiograms of Daily Runners," *South African Medical Journal*, 1970, 44:3-5.

Maganzini, Herman C., "Heat Adaptation and Injury in Football Players," *Maryland State Medical Journal*, 1967, 16:45-49.

Meador, Blake W., "Diving and Medicine," *Virginia Medical Monthly*, 1967, 94:708-710.

Raunio, Hertta; V.-M. Anttonen; P. Savola; and L. Pyykönen, "Notching in the QRS Complex in the Electrocardiogram of Sportsmen," *Annals of Clinical Research*, 1969, 1:5-12.

Rose, Kenneth D., "Measure of an Individual's Athletic Potential by Cardiopulmonary Response to Exercise," *Medical Times,* 1969, 97: 210-219.

Rose, Kenneth D.; F. Lowell Dunn; and Dennis Bargen, "Serum Electrolyte Relationship to Electrocardiographic Change in Exercising Athletes," *Journal of the American Medical Association,* 1966, 195:155-158.

Schreiner, H.R., "Advances in Decompression Research," *Journal of Occupational Medicine,* 1969, 11:229-237.

Shephard, Roy J., "The Heart and Circulation under Stress of Olympic Conditions," *Journal of the American Medical Association,* 1968, 205: 775-779.

Spence, Dale W., "Techniques for Telemetering Biopotentials from Track Athletes during Competition," *Research Quarterly,* 1969, 40: 427-430.

Stiles, Merritt H., "Altitude and Skiing," *The Journal of the Maine Medical Association,* 1971, 62:139-141.

Stockholm, Alan; and Harold H. Morris, "A Baseball Pitcher's Heart Rate during Actual Competition," *Research Quarterly,* 1969, 40:645-649.

Wyndham, C.H.; and W.P. Leary, "Physiological Problems Expected at the Mexico City Olympic Games," *South African Medical Journal,* 1966, 40:985-987.

PREFACE

The physiological effects of exercise on the heart, lungs, and metabolism of normal individuals is the subject of the third volume in this new series. Recent studies which evaluate an athlete's potential by measuring cardio-vascular responses to exercise are included as well as the biopotentials of the human body to withstand the lung pressure experienced during such sports as diving, skiing, and running in high-altitude areas. Also provided are papers which explore the effects of exercise on thyroxin release. Heat adaptation and the relation of sweat gland performance to heat stroke are then discussed in a later section.

Physiology of the Athlete

Measure of an Individual's Athletic Potential By Cardiopulmonary Response to Exercise

Kenneth D. Rose, M.D.

I HAVE been given the responsibility of discussing the measure of an individual's athletic potential by cardiopulmonary response to exercise. The word "potential" implies a pre-existing state holding promise for good, poor, or indifferent capability for future athletic prowess. Furthermore, it implies that this potential is measurable by cardiopulmonary response to exercise, from which measurement a prognostication can be made. This would seem to be a clear-cut, straight-forward responsibility on the face of it until the variables

Supported by the University of Nebraska Research Council and Grant #HE-06204 from the United States Public Health Service.

Presented at American Academy of Orthopedic Surgeons' Post-Graduate Course on Sports Medicine, Oklahoma City, July 30, 1968.

are examined. It then becomes apparent that forecasting athletic potential from cardiopulmonary measurements is quite a complex task. First the sport must be specified since requirements vary between sports and, in fact, within the confines of one sport. Since emphasis is to be on cardiopulmonary response to exercise, it can be assumed however that endurance sports should hold primary interest. Secondly, even endurance sports have subrequirements which make valid prognostications in one invalid in another. Thirdly, cardiopulmonary fitness does not assure neuromuscular skill, strength, nor motivation, all of which are basic requirements for athletic excellence.[1] Lastly, the physical state of a subject can be modified by training or lack of it so that any given measurement reflects the current situation and not necessarily the end state. Thus, the task of assessing athletic potential is not amenable to easy solution.

Johnson[2] stated in 1946 that "Quantitative assessment of physical fitness is one of the most complex and controversial problems in applied physiology." According to Shephard[3] the situation has not changed much since then. This is true in spite of the sophistication in testing equipment and procedures attending the electronic era. Physical fitness has been described as "the ability of the organism to maintain the various internal equilibria as closely as possible to the resting state during strenuous exertion and to restore promptly, after exercise, any equilibrium which has been disturbed."[4] In order to test physical fitness, it is necessary to describe conditions as to time, duration, and intensity of exercise stress.[3] The purpose of a cardiovascular fitness test, therefore, should be to determine (1) how the heart and vascular system meet augmented metabolism from specified physical stress and (2) whether the coronary circulation is adequate for the increased myocardial metabolism.[5] To be of practical value, a fitness test should be first capable of providing information to serve both purposes yet be simple enough to permit widespread usage[5] and secondly to be so standardized as to permit reproducibility with accuracy.

Good tests of cardiopulmonary fitness are available and applicable but unfortunately, to my knowledge, none have been applied in a long-term study to assess potential for athletic capability. Ideally, one would hope to start with a virgin population assessing their cardiopulmonary fitness and then, by long-term controlled follow-up studies, determine which developed into excellent athletes and which did not. Only under these circumstances could cardiopulmonary fitness truly be used to assess athletic potential.

Powell[6] recently compiled an index of most of the research in track and field sports between 1900-1963. Some of his conclusions are revealing:

1. "So much of the writing in track and field has been based solely on conjecture and opinion, it has been difficult to identify what is empirically believed and what has been scientifically founded and proved."

2. "The only subject concerning an actual event to have received more than cursory attention is the sprint start, its relation to action and subsequent speed in running."

3. "Many mechanical and predictive analyses were initially conceived in the 1930 era, but only three have been located dated later than 1940."

Thus, out of the 372 studies reported by this author, only three since 1940 have been concerned, even remotely, with predictive analysis, and Powell implies that even these are difficult to analyze objectively. Here, then, is an unexplored area for investigation. Is it possible, on the basis of physiological and psychological analysis, to predict the future athletic potential of any young man or woman? As yet this has not been done. Perhaps the reason is that natural selection slowly sifts the gifted from the non-gifted leaving only those hereditarily, psychologically and physically endowed with attributes necessary for superiority. The remainder drop by the wayside. This is a natural, effective and common means for identifying athletic potential although time consuming. We abhor trial and error methods, however, and seek an easy, predictive procedure, presumably so that maximum training effort can be expended on the gifted.

Over the years, many tests of cardiovascular fitness have been proposed, tested on athletes as against non-athletes, and advanced as means whereby those with athletic potential might be identified. Among those are the brachial pulse wave test of Cureton and others, the Q-first heart sound test of Hyman, the oxygen pulse of Holloman, the cardiopulmonary index of Dr. Hyman and others, and, of course, the Harvard step test and its multitude of modifications. They are listed in Table 1.

TABLE 1

Physiological Tests of Cardiopulmonary Excellence

Heart Weight, Size and Volume[7-10]	Cardiopulmonary Index[19]
Ballistocardiography[11]	Serum Electrolytes[20]
Roentgenkymography[12]	Electrocardiography [21-23]
Oxygen—Pulse[12]	Lactate Production[24]
Brachial Pulse Wave[13]	Maximum Oxygen
Q-First Heart Sound[14]	Consumption[25]
Step Tests—	Bicycle Ergometer[26]
Pulse Rates[15-18]	Treadmill Tests[27, 28]
	Walk—Run Tests[29, 30]

Applied in comparative studies of trained vs. untrained subjects, they all demonstrate the better cardiopulmonary fitness and oxygen utilization so characteristic of the trained athlete. Many of these depend upon submaximal heart rate as part of the formula for calculation of fitness. It is an accepted fact that any isolated heart rate of any individual, at any time, is subject to considerable variability brought about by ingestion of food, external temperature and humidity, state of training, emotional state, etc. such that tests relying on submaximal heart rate suffer from this inborn error. Furthermore, submaximal and even maximal heart rate is so variable by age that valid interage comparisons are impossible. (Figure 1) Other tests, such as the Q-first heart sound, brachial pulse wave analysis, and heart size and weight have at best a tenuous relationship to fitness. Recovery tests such as the step tests and electrocardiogram changes relate to the ability of the cardiovascular system to re-establish homeostasis at a level approaching the resting state and are frequently a victim of external variables. For that reason, exercise physiologists have come to rely upon maximum oxygen consumption per kilogram body weight as the least equivocal method for approaching valid comparison between subjects, on which all predictive analyses must be made.[3]

The maximum oxygen consumption test is based on simple physiological facts. Increase in heart rate and oxygen consumption attend onset of exercise, both increasing linearly to a plateau beyond which further increase in work output results in no further increase in either oxygen utilization or pulse rate.[25] This level of oxygen consumption is termed "maximum oxygen consumption," a value which, for all practical purposes, reflects the individual's aerobic

FIGURE 1

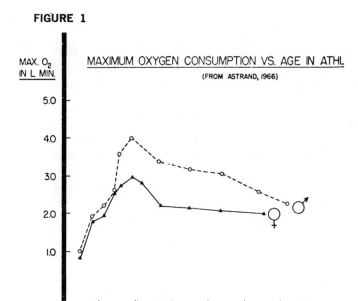

MAX. O$_2$ IN L MIN.

MAXIMUM OXYGEN CONSUMPTION VS. AGE IN ATHL

(FROM ASTRAND, 1966)

AGE

power or his ability to take in oxygen, distribute it, and use it effectively at the tissue level. The test can be done either with a bicycle ergometer as a stressing device, after the method of Astrand,[26] or with a treadmill after the method of Bruce[28] and others. Oxygen consumption is continuously monitored. The

TABLE 2

(Adapted from Taylor, 1966)

Maximal Oxygen Intake in Ml. Per Kilogram of Body Weight

Subjects	No.	Ml./Kg.
Students (Untrained)	68	42-65
Soldiers	24	50-55
Students (Intramural)	7	54-60
Varsity Football	10	58-66
Varsity Track	15	64-74
Don Lash*	1	81

* Data of Robinson, Edwards and Dill.

stress of riding an ergometer is independent of body weight, and subjects usually tire before reaching cardiopulmonary maximum. Thus, maximum oxygen consumption data, based on ergometry, do not reach the magnitude of those employing a treadmill. This is a valid argument for use of the latter procedure.

Data on maximum oxygen consumption in young adults, adapted from Taylor's work, are shown in Table 2. Here it is seen that consumption in milliliters per kilogram of body weight per minute varies from a low of 42 in untrained, normal students to a high of 74 milliliters in trained trackmen. Of considerable importance, in terms of predictive value, is the overlap between non-athletic students and athletes. A 64 milliliter maximum oxygen consumption in a non-athletic male student implies that that individual is endowed with a cardiopulmonary system capable of almost any degree of sustained effort. Cooper[31] has empirically observed non-athletic Air Force recruits with intrinsically high maximum oxygen consumptions, a capability which was apparently hereditary and not the result of a sustained exercise program. It may be that the high values recorded for athletes in Table 2 reflect the net result of the natural winnowing process mentioned earlier. If this is the case, maximum oxygen consumption determinations done in early adolescence may in truth give a cardiopulmonary clue to future athletic prowess. Dr. Bailey reported on the initial phases of such a study at the University of Saskatchewan in 1966.[32] Later data apparently are not available. More such studies, of course, are needed.

But treadmills and oxygen monitoring equipment are costly and not always available. It has been necessary to seek other, less complicated means for assessing cardiopulmonary fitness. The most recent and best one to appear

TABLE 3
Cooper's Physical Fitness Category

Fitness Category	Distance Covered	Oxygen Consumption
I Very poor	less than 1.0 mile	28.0 ml's or less
II Poor	1.0 to 1.24 miles	28.1 to 34 ml's
III Fair	1.25 to 1.49 miles	34.1 to 42 ml's
IV Good	1.50 to 1.74 miles	42.1 to 52 ml's
V Excellent	1.75 miles or more	52.1 ml's or more

in the literature is Cooper's 12-minute walk-run test.[33] An offshoot of Balke's 11-minute walk-run test, and one which has been documented by concomitant oxygen consumption studies, it has enjoyed a meteoric rise in popularity by virtue of its association with his "Aerobics" exercise program. Table 3, extracted from his book, presents the details of fitness assessment. The University of Nebraska football team was tested by this method during spring football practice. The "excellent" category was reached by 4.0%, 54% were classified "good" while 42% were either "fair" or "poor." By the end of spring practice this had changed so that now 28.7% were in the "excellent" and 63.8% were in the "good" category while only 7.3% were now in "fair" or "poor." Even though there was a wide divergence of results between the varsity team members, who is to say that all below 52 ml. per kilogram per minute were not excellent athletes?

Athletes do vary in their cardiopulmonary competence. Recently we completed a three-year study of serum electrolyte and radiotelemetered electrocardiographic variables in untrained students vs. trained varsity trackmen. This was reported, in part, here last year.[34] Figure 2 presents this data for serum calcium along with the data for Charlie Green, one of the world's fastest sprint men. Mr. Green, who had never before run a 440 yard dash and who had devoted most of his training time to perfecting his fantastic capability for the rapid start, ran a 48.3 second 440 yard dash wearing a 28 ounce transmitter. His serum calcium increase exceeded the values of the 52 untrained subjects and, by far, the values of the trained distance runner. His telemetered electrocardiogram is shown in Figure 3 along with that of a trained varsity mile runner. Characteristic of the well-trained track runner is the steep T-wave, increasing with exercise. Mr. Green's was flat and with little post exercise change. Mr. Green was also bothered considerably with muscle cramps and nausea after the race. The flat T-waves, the high calcium response to exercise and the post-race cramps and nausea are all signs of lack of what is rec-

FIGURE 2

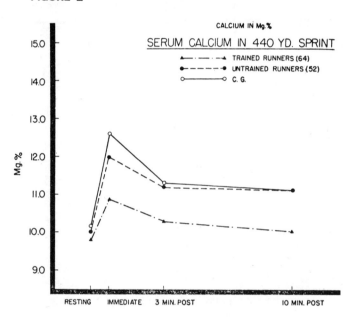

ognized as physical fitness. No one, however, would say that Charlie Green does not possess athletic prowess by virtue of it. If there is some doubt of it, observe his record and his action in the 1968 Olympics.

Runners such as Mr. Green are the exception rather than the rule, however, when it comes to amplitude of the pre-cordial T-wave. The high amplitude standard T-wave or bipolar telemetered ECG are so characteristic of the athlete who has devoted much of his adolescent and young adult life to hard endurance training they are almost pathognomonic. Tuttle

FIGURE 3

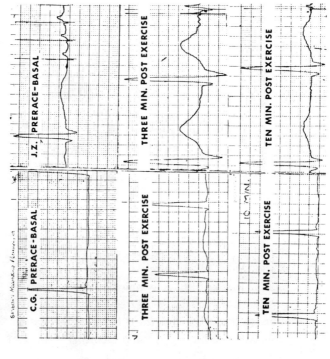

Radiotelemetered E.C.G. of sprint (C.G.) and distance (J.Z.) runners before and after 440 yard dash.*

* Standardized to 1 mv. and recorded at 95 mm/sec.

20

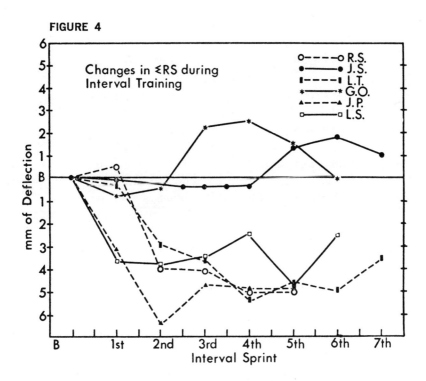

FIGURE 4

Changes in ≤RS during Interval Training

○----○ R.S.
●——● J.S.
▮----▮ L.T.
＊——＊ G.O.
▲----▲ J.P.
□——□ L.S.

mm of Deflection

B 1st 2nd 3rd 4th 5th 6th 7th
Interval Sprint

TABLE 4

T-Wave Recovery Times After

Interval Running*

Subject	Training	T-Wave Recovery Time (Min.)	Coach's Rating
L.T.	2 mo.	3	Good
L.T.	4 mo.	3	Good
R.S.	5 mo.	5	Good
L.S.	2 mo.	8	Good
J.P.	2 mo.	9	Good
A.O.	2 mo.	14	Fair-Poor
D.S.	1 mo.	16	Poor
D.C.	6 mo.	18	Fair
J.S.	2 mo.	20	Fair
W.C.	5 mo.	20	Fair

*5 or 6-440 yard sprints with interval 220 yard jogs.

21

and Karns[35] reported observing increases in T-wave amplitude in athletes after a season of training and Carlisle and Carlisle[21] observed striking changes in T-amplitude with training and overtraining. We followed the resting and post 220 yard dash telemetered bi-axial electrocardiogram on 15 high school track athletes for three years, from the beginning of the sophomore through the end of the senior year. No electrocardiographic changes of any kind were observed, with the exception of the disappearance of post-exercise supraventricular extrasystoles in one boy following a year of training. Certainly, no presence of nor development of the traditional high amplitude T-waves, such as appear in Figure 3, were noted, suggesting that this type of ECG pattern is a result of prolonged intensive training and has no predictive value.

TABLE 5
Work Pulse Rates of Athletes Before and After Procedural Adaptation*

Subject	First Trial	After Adaptation	Change
Fi	151	123	−28
JJ	139	116	−23
Gi	142	130	−12
CB	135	137	+ 2
CP	121	121	0
DH	128	125	− 3
RR	137	138	+ 1

* As adapted from Taylor's data.

Although the maximum oxygen consumption test is undoubtedly the best measure of cardiopulmonary fitness, other methods of assessing such fitness need not be neglected. Observing variations in the rate at which the post-race electrocardiogram returned to its resting configuration, specifically the time required of the T-wave of the electrocardiogram to first return of its pre-race amplitude, this "T-wave recovery time" was compared to athletic prowess in 10 varsity distance runners.

The coaches' rating is compared to electrocardiogram recovery time in Table 4. Admittedly a brief and inconclusive study, it does indirectly reveal decided variations, even in varsity athletes in rate of recovery from the marked oxygen debt attending the running of a strenuous sprint race.

The telemetered electrocardiogram reveals other unusual variables related to fitness. The sum of the amplitudes of the R and S wave of the electrocardiogram decrease considerably below resting measurements in the well-trained athlete. In Figure 4, data are presented

FIGURE 5

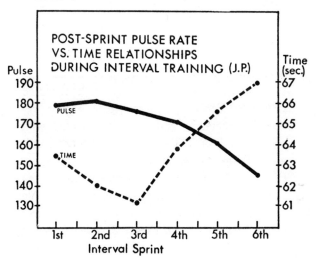

FIGURE 6

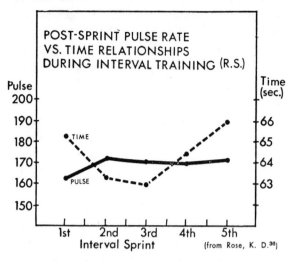

POST-SPRINT PULSE RATE
VS. TIME RELATIONSHIPS
DURING INTERVAL TRAINING (R.S.)

(from Rose, K. D.[36])

for four top-rated and two low-rated distance runners. The values represent sums of the R and S wave amplitudes greater or less than resting (B) using each subject's resting measurement as his control. The difference between the two groups is obvious. Whether this observation will stand up under a large population study is now being investigated. Nevertheless, this interesting indirect measurement of cardiac function has some value in assessing cardiopulmonary fitness in relation to athletic capability.

Fitness tests based on pulse rate may be invalidated by the learning process, lack of motivation, decreased anxiety with repeated tests, etc. Table 5, adapted from Taylor, reveals decreases in pulse rate associated with repeated treadmill tests. Such errors are eliminated if the subject can reach true maximum exertion. Even in treadmill maximum oxygen consumption tests, such an error is possible when the subject, through anxiety, stops short of his true maximum. Figure 5 shows how the

24

FIGURE 7

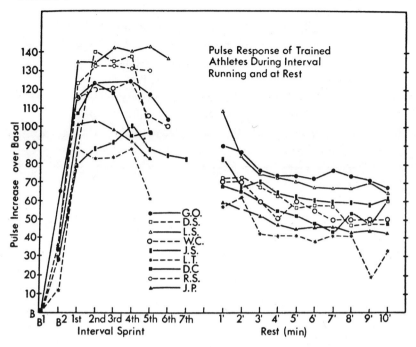

Pulse Response of Trained
Athletes During Interval
Running and at Rest

Pulse Increase over Basal

Legend:
—●— G.O.
---□--- D.S.
—△— L.S.
---○--- W.C.
—■— J.S.
---■--- L.T.
—■— D.C
---○--- R.S.
—▲— J.P.

x-axis: B, B1, B2, 1st 2nd 3rd 4th 5th 6th 7th — Interval Sprint; 1' 2' 3' 4' 5' 6' 7' 8' 9' 10' — Rest (min)

telemetered heart rate can detect such decline
in motivation in a runner doing 440 yard
sprints interspersed with 220 yard jogs. Figure 6[36] is a similar study in a tiring runner.
His heart rate stayed constant but his times
increased. Data in Figure 7 are from an inter-
val-run study of nine distance runners and
reveal some interesting facts. B1 is the true
resting pulse for each subject and represents
his zero point. B2 reflects pulse increases following application of the electrodes and the
radiotransmitter. The remainder revealed pulse
rate increases, over resting level, immediately
following each 440 yard sprint. Note the 12-65
beat increase folowing the radio attachment.
This is pure anxiety and, in the case of GO,
50% of the total pulse increase even with exercise. Also note the wide divergence in total

25

pulse increase, the range being 90-140 beats per minute. What does this tell us? It tells us that measure of state of training or athletic capability based on resting pulse, pulse increase following exercise, and decrease following cessation of exercise is an individual thing, widely variable, influenced by anxiety, dependent on degree of effort, and difficult to standardize. Thus, this commonly used field method for assessing athletic fitness is subject to too many errors to make it of practical value.

Summary

I would like to summarize, briefly, the points presented in the foregoing discussion. Several things are apparent. First, it is possible to equate cardiopulmonary fitness with athletic ability. It stands to reason that anyone with good or excellent cardiovascular response most likely possesses other physical capabilities compatible with athletic excellence. It must be added, however, that this statement is more true concerning endurance sports than strength or skill sports. Secondly, the best cardiovascular fitness tests are treadmill tests to determine maximum aerobic capacity. Their pre-eminence comes from their ease of standardization. When properly applied, maximum aerobic capacity tests bypass most of the artifacts inherent in fitness tests. It should be added, however, that they do have a limitation, this being the motivation factor. Thirdly, in spite of possible artifacts in brachial pulse analysis, exercise and recovery electrocardiography, Q-first heart sound measurements, breath-holding tests, etc., it would be scientifically nearsighted to discount them as research tools for the study of fitness. Fourthly, electrocardiographic changes, cardiac anatomical variations, bradycardia and increased stroke volume, etc., of the fit, endurance athlete probably takes many years to develop, and thus these measures, per se, cannot be used in early assessment of athletic capability. Lastly, practicality dictates wider use of exercise tests such as Balke's and Cooper's walk-run tests. Prospective studies are needed to equate cardiovascular pulmonary fitness in early life with future athletic prowess. Dr. Cooper has initiated such a study, and with his population, USAF regulars, he stands a good chance of reaching an early answer to the question. Dr. Bailey, who has and presumably still is studying young children in terms of their maximum oxygen consumption, may in time also arrive at an early answer. Until such studies become available, physical fitness tests of all kinds can really be applied only to demonstrate an already well-known fact, namely, well-trained, capable athletes possess a much better cardiovascular pulmonary system than those of their less fit and untrained counterparts.

Bibliography

1. Jokl, E.: Heart and Sports, Charles C. Thomas, Springfield, 1964, p. 3.

2. Johnson, H. E.: Applied Physiology, Ann. Rev. Physiol. 8: 535-558 (1946).

3. Shephard, R. J.: Physiological Determinants of Cardiopulmonary Fitness, Jour. Sports Med and Phys. Fitness 7: 111-134 (Sept.) 1967.

4. Darling, R. C.: The Significance of Physical Fitness, Arch. Physical Med. 28: 140-145 (1947).

5. Bruce, R. A., Rowell, L. B., Blackmon, J. R. and Doan, A.: Cardiovascular Function Tests, The Heart Bulletin 14: 9-14 (1965).

6. Powell, J. T.: A Compilation and Analysis of Classified Indexed and/or Completed Research in Track and Field Athletics, Coaching Review 5: 7-12 (June) 1967.

7. Karvonen, M. J.: Effects of Vigorous Exercise on the Heart: In Work and the Heart. Edited by Rosenbaum, F. F. and Belknap, E. L., Paul E. Hoeber, New York, 1959.

8. Mellerowicz, H.: Cited in Jokl, E. op cit, p. 26.

9. Jokl, E. et al: Sports in the Cultural Pattern of the World, Institute of Occupational Health, Helsinki, 1956.

10. Cureton, T. K.: Physical Fitness of Champion Athletes, U. III. Press, Urbana, 1951, pp. 105-136.

11. Jokl, E.: Ballistocardiographic Studies on Athletes, Amer. Jour. Cardiology 4: 105-117 (July) 1959.

12. Reindell, H.: Cited in Jokl, E., Heart and Sports, Ibid, pp. 29-35.

13. Cureton, T. K., Ibid.

14. Hyman, A. S.: The Q-First Heart Sound Interval in Athletes at Rest and after Exercise, Jour. Sports Med. and Phys. Fitness 4: 199-203 (Dec.) 1964.

15. Gallagher, J. R. and Brouha, L.: V. A Simple Method for Evaluating Fitness in Boys: The Step Test, Yale Jour. Biol. and Med. 15: 769-779 (July) 1943.

16. Astrand, P. O. and Rhyming, I.: A Nomogram for Calculation of Aerobic Capacity (Physical Fitness) from Pulse Rate during Submaximal Work. Jour. Applied Physiol. 8: 73-80 (1965).

17. Tuttle, W. W.: The Use of the Pulse-Ratio Test for Rating Physical Efficiency, Res. Quarterly 2: 5-17 (1931).

18. Karvonen, M. J., Ibid.

19. Hyman, A. S.: Physical Fitness and Heart Disease, Medical Times 93: 284-289 (Mar.) 1965.

20. Rose, K. D. and Dunn, F. L.: A Study of Heart Function in Athletes by Telemetered Electrocardiography, Proc. 5th Nat. Conf. Med. Aspects Sports, AMA, Chicago, 1963, pp. 30-36.

21. Carlisle, F. and Carlisle, U.: Physiological Studies of Australian Olympic Swimmers in Hard Training, Australian Jour. Physical Ed. 23: 5-34 (1961).

22. Rose, K. D., Dunn, F. L. and Bargen, D.: Serum Electrolyte Relationship to Electrocardiographic Change in Exercising Athletes, Jour. Amer. Med. Ass'n. 195: 111-114 (Jan.) 1966.

23. Cureton, T. K., Ibid., pp. 137-227.

24. Margaria, R., Edwards, H. T. and Dill, D. B.: The Possible Mechanism of Contracting. and Paying the Oxygen Debt and the Role of Lactic Acid in Muscular Contraction, Amer. Jour. Physiol. 106: 689 (1933).

25. Taylor, H. L., Buskirk, E. and Henschel, A.: Maximum Oxygen Intake as an Objective Measure of Cardiorespiratory Performance, Jour. Applied Physiol. 8: 73-80 (1955).

26. Astrand, Per-Olof: Work Tests with the Bicycle Ergometer, Monark, Varberg, Sweden.

27. Balke, B.: Correlation of Static and Physical Endurance. I. A Test of Physical Performance Based on the Cardiovascular and Respiratory Responses to Gradually increased Work. Report No. 1, Project No. 21-32-004, Randolph Air Force Base, Tex.: USAF School of Aerospace Med., (April) 1952.

28. Bruce, R. A., et al, Ibid.

29. Balke, B.: A Simple Field Test for the Assessment of Physical Fitness. CARI REPORT 63-18, Oklahoma City: Civil Aeromedical Research Institute, Federal Aviation Agency, (Sept.) 1963.

30. Cooper, K. H.: Aerobics, M. Evans and Co. and J. B. Lippincott, New York, Philadelphia, 1968, pp. 44-55.

31. Cooper, K. H.: Personal Communication, (1968).

32. Bailey, D. A. and Orban, A. R.: Monitoring all Outwork by Radiotelemetry. Presented at Amer. Coll. Sports Med. Ann. Meeting, Hollywood, Calif., Mar. 20, 1964.

33. Cooper, K. H.: USAF Physical Fitness Program, AFP # 50-40 (Test) Dept. of the Air Force, Washington, D. C., (Mar.) 1968.

34. Rose, K. D.: Telemetry in the Study of the Heart in Athletes, Part II. Proc. Post Graduate Course on Sports Medicine, Amer. Acad. Orth. Surg., Oklahoma City, 1967, C. V. Mosby, St. Louis (in press).

35. Tuttle, W. W. and Korns, H. M.: Electrocardiographic Observations on Athletes· before and after Season of Physical Training, Amer. Heart Jour. 21: 104-107 (Jan.) 1941.

36. Rose, K. D.: Telemetry in the Study of the Heart in Athletes. Part I, Proc. Post-Graduate Course on Sports Medicine, American Academy of Orthopedic Surgeons, C. V. Mosby, St. Louis (in press).

Serum Electrolyte Relationship to Electrocardiographic Change in Exercising Athletes

Kenneth D. Rose, MD, F. Lowell Dunn, MD, and Dennis Bargen

Increase in amplitude and peaking of the T wave of the electrocardiogram following exercise is a well-known phenomenon. It was first reported in 1908 by Muller and Nicholai,[1] and their observations have been frequently confirmed in the following years.[2,3] The peaked precordial T wave associated with the immediate postexercise period is essentially identical with T wave in hyperkalemia. However, very little effort has been made to correlate the two, although there have been numerous well-documented reports linking physical exercise to transient increases in serum and plasma potassium levels.[4] Since Fenn's[5,6] excellent review articles, it has been an accepted fact that potassium efflux from somatic muscle to extracellular space attends contraction, and Grupp,[7] among others, has shown that potassium transfer from the extracellular spaces surrounding muscle cells in situ to the circulating plasma is extremely rapid, if not instantaneous.

Winkler, et al[8] in slow-perfusion experiments with dogs, demonstrated T-wave peaking as the earliest sign of increasing plasma potassium levels,

Read before the 43rd annual meeting of the American College Health Association. Miami Beach, Fla, April 30, 1965.

30

this electrocardiographic change occurring with as little increase as 0.9 mEq/liter.

Kahn and Simonson[3] noted that the precordial T-wave amplitude increases with vigorous treadmill exercise were not due to positional change alone, suggesting they were a reflection of relative, generalized myocardial hypoxia. Their statement that these changes were not associated with variation in serum potassium levels, not supported by data or by a statement as to time of sampling, is difficult to evaluate in the light of the known rapid changes in this electrolyte attending vigorous exercise.[4] Braun et al[9] have studied the precordial hyperkalemic T wave in great detail, describing it as narrow, tall, steep, and pointed (paper speed 25 mm/sec). T waves of this nature are accepted as electrocardiographic evidence of hyperpotassemia.

A report correlating peaked precordial T waves and serum potassium levels during athletic exercise has been made by Beckner and Winsor,[10] whose data suggested to them that the two parameters were not associated. These authors drew blood samples no earlier than eight minutes and at times as long as 35 minutes after exercise (personal communication, Travis Winsor, MD, March 1964), whereas postexercise increase in circulating potassium is transient, lasting two to three minutes at most.[4] Thus, the relationship between strenuous physical effort, the physiological potassium perfusion attending such effort, and peaking of the precordial T wave of the ECG has yet to be elucidated.

Cureton[11] mentioned many years ago that perfection of radio recording of the ECG in athletes might further clarify the exercise T-wave problem. Since then, radiotelecardiography has been perfected, and clinical tracings are possible.[12] Applying this technique, we have been studying the electrocardiographic patterns attending strenuous physical effort by trained distance runners.[13] Since a correlation between stamina and athletic capability in trained distance runners and the rapidity with which their postexercise precordial T wave (CR_5-C_5 lead application) returned to normal was noted, it was suggested that the so-called T-wave recovery time might be an indication of overall cardiopulmonary efficiency. The current report concerns further investigation into the postexercise ECG. It is primarily a study of the relationship between the rapid increase in circulating serum potassium attending exercise and the precordial T wave in an attempt to determine some of the basic facts underlying this phenomenon.

Materials and Methods

The test subjects were all male university students between the ages of 18 and 22, five of whom were fully trained middle-distance and distance runners with several years experience and five of whom were untrained physical-education students. Of the latter group, only one (patient 4) had engaged in a significant amount of athletics in high school, and he had not been involved in a training program for two years.

All were subjected to thorough physical examinations prior to participation, including a chest x-ray film and a double-Master ECG. One (patient 5) was found to have a left parasternal systolic murmur which, on repeated examination by our cardiologist, was judged functional in type. The remainder were free from defect and were considered in excellent physical condition.

The technique of radiotelecardiography has been described in detail in previous publications.[12,13]

Table 1.—Changes in Serum Potassium Levels Attending
Vigorous Exercise and Recovery

Patient	Age, Yr	State of Training	Serum Potassium Level, mEq/Liter			
			Basal	Immediate	3 Min Rest	10 Min Rest
1	21	Untrained	3.9	5.0	3.9	4.6
2	20	Untrained	4.6	5.9	3.7	4.0
3	20	Untrained	4.0	5.3	4.0	4.0
4	20	Untrained	4.4	5.1	3.6	4.0
5	20	Untrained	4.9	5.5	4.0	4.3
6	22	Trained	3.7	4.8	3.6	3.8
7	18	Trained	3.9	5.3	3.9	3.8
8	23	Trained	4.1	5.4	3.5	3.9
9	22	Trained	4.2	6.1	4.4	3.9
10	18	Trained	4.3	5.5	3.9	3.9

Briefly, it comprises the use of a lightweight AM-FM transmitter carried in a padded belt over the sacrum. Bipolar-biaxillary leads (CR_5-C_5) feed the single precordial information into the transmitter, which transmits it to a remote receiver-filter-recorder complex where the data is recorded for future analysis. Because somatic muscle potentials are similar in frequency to those emanating from the heart, diagnostic ECGs have not been obtained during the actual run. Radiotelemetry, however, makes it possible to record instantaneous tracings during or following exercise, as there is no need to spend time applying leads. In this way, transient changes are recorded which might be missed by use of standard electrocardiographic techniques. The standard tape speed of 25 mm/sec is not fast enough to separate the various components of the ECG at postexercise pulse rates of 160 to 190 beats per minute commonly encountered. Wave analysis is made, however, on tracings recorded at 85 mm/sec. A short burst of recording at slow speed (9.5 mm/sec) permits accurate counting of heart rate and more clearly depicts the traditional "peaked" T-wave form seen following exercise than does the fast recording.

Table 2.—Changes in Serum Sodium Levels Attending Vigorous Exercise and Recovery

Patient	Serum Sodium Level, mEq/Liter				Perspiration After Race
	Basal	Immediate	3 Min Rest	10 Min Rest	
1	146	146	145	144	Excessive
2	140	147	140	140	Minimal
3	136	140	138	139	Minimal
4	146	143	145	136	Minimal
5	140	151	140	144	Excessive
6	141	142	138	137	Excessive
7	139	145	142	136	Minimal
8	147	150	150	145	Excessive
9	140	148	143	140	Excessive
10	137	144	140	140	Minimal

Twelve-milliliter samples of blood were drawn from the antecubital vein immediately preceding and immediately following exercise (within ten seconds) and at three and ten minutes after exercise. The ECG was recorded during venipuncture so that the tracing would reflect the existing serum electrolyte status. The blood was allowed to clot at room temperature for one hour and was spun in a centrifuge at 1,500 rpm for five minutes and the serum separated immediately. Observable hemolysis did not occur. Serum samples were divided into two aliquots, a 2-ml specimen being used for calcium analysis by the Ferro-Hamm technique.[14] Control specimens containing known calcium concentrations were analyzed parallel with each test sample to determine standard deviation of the procedure. ($\pm$0.1 mg/100 ml). Sodium and potassium were analyzed by flame photometry by two independent clinical pathology laboratories, and the results correlated closely. Use of coded specimens obviated bias on the part of the technicians.

Results

Serum potassium.—In every instance there was an increase in circulating serum potassium immediately following exercise, varying from 0.6 to as much as 1.9 mEq/liter (Table 1). In trained subjects the rise averaged 1.38 mEq/liter and in untrained subjects 1 mEq/liter. This was followed by an immediate decrease in levels, averaging 1.56 mEq/liter in trained and 1.52 mEq/liter in untrained subjects, the three-minute levels being 0.18 and 0.52 mEq/liter below resting levels, respective-

Table 3.—Changes in Serum Calcium Levels Attending Vigorous Exercise and Recovery

Patient	Serum Calcium Level, Mg/100 Ml			
	Basal	Immediate	3 Min Rest	10 Min Rest
1	9.8	9.8	9.8	10.0
2	10.4	11.5	12.6	10.0
3	10.0	10.0	10.0	10.7
4	10.0	9.8	9.6	9.8
5	9.8	12.0	10.2	....
6	9.6	9.8	11.1	10.4
7	11.9	10.0	12.2	11.5
8	9.3	10.4	10.9	10.4
9	9.3	11.5	10.0	10.0
10	10.2	12.5	11.5	10.9

ly. In both groups, the potassium levels ten minutes after exercise were approximately 0.2 mEq/liter below the resting values. There was an increase in the amplitude of the T waves after exercise, with one exception. This increase was more noticeable in the trained than in the untrained subjects. Decline in the T-wave

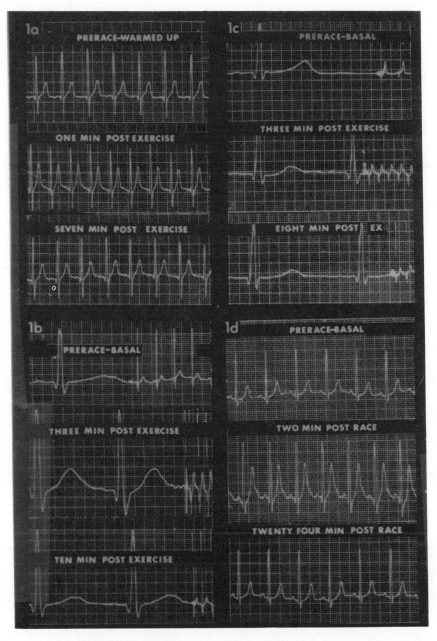

Radiotelecardiographic patterns in exercise and recovery (*a*, patient 6; *b*, patient 10; *c*, patient 4; *d*, patient 11).

amplitude to preexercise level was consistently delayed several minutes after the serum potassium level had returned to near basal value.

A representative series of tracings is shown in the accompanying Figure.

The bipolar CR_5-C_5 lead ECG after exercise presents a heterogeneous pattern of primary and secondary T-wave changes. Figure 1a, recorded at standard speed, shows a primary T-wave amplitude increase; 1b is probably a complex mixture of both; while 1c, from an untrained subject, reveals a 2-mm decrease in T-wave amplitude after exercise. Figure 1d, the ECG of a patient not included in the study, was also recorded at standard speed and is an example of obvious primary T-wave peaking and increase in amplitude caused by intense effort. Although the single-lead telemetered ECG is unable to identify primary T-wave changes consistently in all subjects, experience has shown that postexercise variations in the electrocardiographic pattern cannot be explained on the basis of ventricular gradient alone, and some additional factor must be postulated.

Serum Sodium.—Serum sodium levels did not change to any noticeable degree (Table 2). Although Wit and Dalderup[15] had observed an increase in sodium following prolonged exercise and had concluded that this was the result of fluid loss through perspiration, no such correlation existed here. Record was kept of subjects who perspired heavily and those who did not. No consistent relationship existed between this sign of fluid loss and increased sodium levels. The 440-yard race requires only 50 to 65 seconds, and little time is available for significant dehydration.

Serum Calcium.—Calcium values following exercise varied erratically, and at times considerably beyond the procedural error of ±0.1 mg/100 ml. There was no apparent explanation for the variations in the range of 2.2 mg/100 ml which occurred in five of the subjects (Table 3).

Comment

The results presented here support the findings of others who have studied exercise-induced changes in serum potassium,[4-6] and also demonstrate that the earliest electrocardiographic sign of increased circulating potassium levels (peaking and increased amplitude of the T wave) can occur following rapid rate of change in its ionic level. The data further show that, in healthy, young college males, the concentrations of sodium and calcium change erratically or not at all with brief, vigorous exercise and that these ions probably play little if any part in the concurrent electrocardiographic wave-amplitude variations.

Unanswered is whether the observed potassium ion changes do, in fact, cause the primary T-wave changes. That this factor must be considered is suggested by the work of Winkler et al[8] with dogs, of Keith et al[16] with humans, and of others, all of whom demonstrated T-wave peaking with artificially, slowly induced hyperkalemia. Ladé and Brown[17] and Brown and Goot,[18] by showing that respiratory acidosis, such as that caused by muscular work, enhances potassium shift from somatic to cardiac muscle, have contributed to an understanding of this physiological process, as has Grupp,[7] who reported an increased influx of potassium into heart muscle associated with potassium perfusion and increased heart rates. Our experience[19] with spectators at football games and those of Roman[20] with F100-F jet pilots practicing low-level infiltration bombing runs, whose ECGs showed pronounced tachycardia but no peaked T waves, indicate that tachycardia-induced positional changes play no part in the development of the high-amplitude, peaked T wave.

The T waves attending short-term, vigorous exercise become maximum within a minute or two after exercise and decline slowly during the succeeding few minutes. That they do not precisely follow the blood potassium level, which is basal or subbasal by three minutes after exercise, may be due to slow potassium washout, following cessation of physiological perfusion.[7] We have postulated[13] that the time required for the T wave to return to basal level after exercise is a function of cardiopulmonary efficiency and that rapid rates of return are characteristic of the fully trained athlete, and we have presented some data to support this. Grupp's[7] observation that the rate of myocardial potassium efflux was proportional to coronary flow would tend to support this postulate.

Summary

Postexercise peaking and amplitude increase of the precordial T wave of the electrocardiogram resembles that observed in the hyperkalemia of disease or experimental potassium feeding or perfusion. Transient increase in serum potassium level is known to follow muscular effort. Five trained and five untrained male subjects, 18 to 22 years of age, were used in a study to determine the possible relationship between serum sodium, potassium, and calcium levels and electrocardiographic changes as determined by radiotelecardiography. No significant or consistent variations were observed in sodium or calcium levels, but immediate postexercise potassium levels increased by 0.6 to 1.9 mEq/liter. There was an associated, transient increased amplitude of the precordial T wave, greater in the trained than in the untrained subjects. This observation is explained on the basis of a physiological potassium perfusion resulting from intensive muscular effort.

This investigation was supported by Public Health Service grant HE-06402 from the National Heart Institute.

References

1. Muller and Nicholai: Effect of Exercise on T-Waves, *Zentralbl Physiologie* 22:58, 1908. quoted by Katz, L.N.: The Significance of the T-Wave in the Electrogram and Electrocardiogram, *Physiol Rev* 8:447-500 (Oct) 1928.

2. Hartwell, A.A., et al: Effect of Exercise and of Four Commonly Used Drugs on Normal Human Electrocardiograms With Particular Reference to T-Wave Changes, *J Clin Invest* 21:409-417 (July) 1942.

3. Kahn, K.A., and Simonson, E.: Changes in Mean Spatial QRS and T-Vectors and of Conventional Electrocardiographic Items in Hard Anaerobic Work, *Circ Res* 5:629-633 (Nov) 1957.

4. DeLanne, R.; Barnes, J.R.; and Brouha, L.: Changes in Osmotic Pressure and Ionic Concentrations of Plasma During Muscular Work and Recovery, *J Appl Physiol* 14:804-808 (May) 1959.

5. Fenn. W.O.: Electrolytes in Muscle, *Physiol Rev* 16:450-487 (July) 1936.

6. Fenn, W.O.: The Role of Potassium in Physiological Processes, *Physiol Rev* 20:377-415 (July) 1940.

7. Grupp, G.: Potassium Exchange in the Dog Heart in Situ, *Circ Res* 13:279-289 (Oct) 1963.

8. Winkler, A.W.; Hoff, H.E.; and Smith, P.K.: Electrocardiographic Changes and Concentration of Potassium in Serum Following Intravenous Injection of Potassium Chloride, *Amer J Physiol* 124:478-483 (Nov) 1938.

9. Braun, H.A.; Surawicz, B.; and Bellet, S.: T-Waves in Hyperpotassemia: Their Differentiation From Simulating T-Waves in Other Conditions, *Amer J Med Sci* 230:147-156 (Aug) 1955.

10. Beckner, G.S., and Winsor, T.: Cardiovascular Adaptation to Prolonged Physical Effort, *Circulation* 9:835-846 (June) 1954.

11. Cureton, T.K., Jr.: Effects of Longitudinal Physical Training on the Amplitude of the Highest Precordial T-Wave of the ECG, *Med Sportiva* 12:259-281 (July) 1958.

12. Rose, K.D.: "Telemetering Physiologic Data From Athletes," in *Proceedings 1965 International Telemetering Conference*, Pasadena, Calif: F. G. McGavock Associates, 1965, pp 225-241.

13. Rose, K.D., and Dunn, F.L.: "A Study of Heart Function in Athletes by Telemetered Electrocardiography," in *Proceedings of the Fifth Annual Conference on Medical Aspects of Sports*, Chicago: American Medical Assoc., 1963, pp 30-37.

14. Ferro, P.V., and Hamm, A.B.: A Simple Spectrophotometric Method for the Determination of Calcium, *Amer J Clin Path* 28:208-217 (Aug) 1957.

15. Wit, A.G.; Dalderup, L.M.; and Pol, G.: Muscular Work and Potassium Supply, *Acta Physiol Pharmacol Neerl* 11:405-410 (March) 1962.

16. Keith, N.H.; Osterberg, A.E.; and Burchell, H.B.: Some Effects of Potassium Salts in Man, *Ann Intern Med* 16:879-892 (May) 1942.

17. Ladé, R., and Brown, E.B., Jr.: Movement of Potassium Between Muscle and Blood in Response to Respiratory Acidosis, *Amer J Physiol* 204:761-764 (May) 1963.

18. Brown, E.B., and Goot, B.: Intracellular Hydrogen Ion Changes and Potassium Movement, *Amer J Physiol* 204:765-770 (May) 1963.

19. Rose, K.D., and Dunn, F.L.: The Heart of the Spectator Sportsman, *Med Times* 92:945-951 (Oct) 1964.

20. Roman, J.A.: Cardiorespiratory Functioning in Flight, *Aerospace Med* 34:322-337 (April) 1963.

The Heart and Circulation Under Stress of Olympic Conditions

Roy J. Shephard, MD, PhD

The nature and extent of the stresses imposed upon the heart and circulation by Olympic competition varies markedly with the type of event. It is thus helpful to make an arbitrary classification of some of the main Olympic contests on the basis of the dominant physiological requirements (Table 1).

The atmosphere of competition imposes an intense psychological stress upon all contestants, and this necessarily acts upon the cardiovascular system. However, psychological stress is greater during anticipation of exercise than during actual performance. Other factors being equal, the cardiovasular effects of psychological stress are thus likely to be greatest in brief repetitive events (categories 4 and 1 of Table 1). All forms of exercise tend to increase the systolic blood pressure. However, certain types of circulatory strain seem related to the mean rather than to the systolic pressure. Elevation of the mean systemic pressure is a particular feature of sustained isometric contractions (such as occur in events from categories 5 and 4 of Table 1). When exercise is sustained for moderately long periods (1 to 60 minutes, events from category 2 of Table 1), the predominant stress is then the maintenance of a maximum cardiac output, with the attendant increase of myocardial metabolism. If exercise is further prolonged (category 3 of Table 1), the circulation is subjected to the additional problems of a cumulative thermal load and a progressive fluid loss.

Inevitably, in any given event there is some overlap between these simple categories, but it is convenient to discuss each separately. The relative stress imposed upon an individual by a specific contest is also influenced by constitutional factors (especially personality and body build), transient variations of bodily status (training, infection, and diet) and interactions with the immediate environment (altitude, heat, air pollution, wind and rain, and the attitude of the spectators).

Psychological Stress

The emotional tachycardia that precedes a race is well-recognized. Åstrand[1] has found pulse rates of 150 beats per minute prior to skiing contests, and British racing drivers awaiting the starter's flag have had pulse rates as high as 200 to 205 beats per minute.[2] In both groups, a tachycardia that was disproportionate to muscular effort recurred when unexpected difficulties were encountered during the event. More detailed physiological studies of the cardiovascular system have yet to be carried out during contests. However, by analogy with laboratory-induced anxiety,[3,4] muscular vasodilation and splanchnic vasoconstriction may be anticipated, with an increase of both cardiac output and mean systemic blood pressure. Furthermore, the pulse rates reported are so high that it is likely that the cardiac stroke volume remains unchanged or is even reduced.

The intensity of the stress imposed upon the heart by an anxiety reaction may exceed that incurred during maximum exercise. This becomes clear from an examination of the nature of cardiac work. The work performed by the ventricle at each pulse beat (W_b) comprises flow and tension components as follows (equation 1):

$$W_b = \int P_v \, dV + \alpha \int P_v \, dt,$$

where P_v is the instantaneous ventricular pressure, V is the ventricular volume, α is a constant related to intramuscular tension, and t is the time over which the tension is maintained. From equation 1, it follows that the work performed per minute by each ventricle is approximated by equation 2:

$$W_t = \bar{P}_v f_h (Q + K),$$

where $\bar{P}_v$ is the mean ventricular pressure, f_h is the heart rate, Q is the stroke volume, and K is a tension factor. Under resting conditions, Kf_h is about thirty times Qf_h, so that the mechanical efficiency of the heart can be as low as 3%[5].

During maximum dynamic exercise, the cardiac output (Qf_h) increases six times; there is a threefold increase of f_h, and a twofold increase of Q. However, the efficiency of the heart increases to 10% to 15%,[5] implying that K has been halved (presumably due to an increased rate of cardiac shortening). The work of the heart is thus increased by only 62%, for a sixfold increase of cardiac output. Let us now contrast this with the situation in the anxious athlete prior to a race. The pulse rate is increased to about the same extent, Q is unchanged, and $\bar{P}_v$ may be increased by 40 mm Hg. Even assuming that K is halved as during exercise (and this is by no means certain), the work of the heart is increased by 114% during the anxiety reaction.

The impact of the increased work load upon the heart muscle depends not only upon the intensity of the work performed, but also upon the adequacy of coronary blood flow relative to work load. The coronary arterial flow occurs mainly during diastole, and tachycardia tends to impede flow by shortening the diastolic phase of the cardiac cycle. Evidence suggesting that anxiety may give rise to myocardial ischemia has been obtained from continuous electrocardiogram recordings on subjects driving in heavy traffic.[2] In athletes with some initial narrowing of the coronary vessels due to congenital or arteriosclerotic disease, it thus seems possible that the additional factor of anxiety could be sufficient to induce a relative ischemia of the myocardium, with infarction and death. I know of no recorded incidents prior to athletic competition. However, the arterial oxygen tension of resting athletes is likely to be substantially lower while they are resident in Mexico City (55 to 60 mm Hg, rather than 80 to 90 mm Hg[6]), and this may conceivably

Table 1.—Categories of Olympic Events, Classified According to Probable Predominant Physiological Requirements

Category 1: Anaerobic Metabolism	Category 2: Aerobic Metabolism	Category 3: Food and Fluid Reserves	Category 4: Explosive Strength	Category 5: Protracted Strength	Category 6: Skill
Running, ≤800 meters	Running, ≥1,000 meters	Marathon	Long jump	Boxing Wrestling	Ballistics Sabre Foil
Swimming, ≤200 meters, 110 meters	Swimming, ≥400 meters, 400 meters	Long-distance cycling	High jump Pole vault	Weight lifting	Sailing Diving
Hurdles	Hurdles Rowing	50-km walk	Throwing javelin, hammer and discus Gymnastics		

precipitate such an episode at the 1968 Olympic Games.

The rise of mean systemic pressure in an anxious contestant also throws a strain upon arteries weakened by congenital or acquired aneurysms. Kirch[7] provides one example of this—a sprint runner who ruptured an aneurysm of the anterior cerebral artery while awaiting the starter's signal.

Many athletes have a very anxious temperament.[8] Perhaps this plays an important role in their success, and, certainly, procedures to diminish anxiety are hard to devise. The cherished warm-up ritual may have some practical value in this connection; the performance of a well-known and familiar routine should reduce anxiety directly, while the peripheral vasodilatation induced by the exercise should minimize the increase of systemic blood pressure.

Isometric Stress

Laboratory experiments have shown that prolonged isometric exercise can give rise to a substantial and progressive increase in the mean systemic blood pressure.[9] This is proportional to the intensity of the isometric contraction (expressed as a percentage of maximum effort for the muscle group concerned), and apparently represents an attempt by the body to maintain perfusion of the active muscle in the face of increasing intramuscular pressure. Intense rhythmic exercise may also lead to some underperfusion of the active muscles during the period of contraction, but while this leads to a progressive increase of systolic pressure, the mean systemic pressure remains relatively unchanged.

No Olympic events require the maintenance of an isometric contraction for the times studied by the physiologists (1 to 5 minutes). On the other hand, the intensities of contraction are greater (100% rather than 50% of the maximum voluntary contraction), and the systemic pressure may be increased by anxiety prior to contraction. Accidents attributable to the rise of mean blood pressure (particularly coronary infarction and vascular rupture) can thus arise following events falling in categories 5 and 4 of Table 1. The hazard is increased by the fact that many weight lifters continue to compete until they are well into the "arteriosclerotic" age range; for instance in the Helsinki Olympics (1952), a quarter of the entrants for the 90-kg weight lifting class were more than 34 years old, and one was 56. In Mexico City, the lowering of the arterial oxygen tension will also increase the likelihood of vascular accidents with isometric exercise.

There would seem to be a case for obtaining more evidence on the extent of dangerous hypertension during such events as weight lifting and wrestling, with a view to possible amendment of rule 40, which states, "There is no age limit for competitors in the Olympic Games." In the meantime, athletes with evidence of arteriosclerosis on fundal examination, hypertension at rest, or abnormalities of the ST-T segment of the ECG taken during exercise should be cautioned against participation in events of this type. Furthermore, it must not be supposed that such episodes are the exclusive prerogative of the middle-aged. Jokl[10] describes a 10-year-old boy who died of "coronary thrombosis" during a boxing match, and a 15-year-old youth who ruptured his aorta after weight lifting.

Endurance Stress

During events having a length of 1 to 60 minutes (category 2), a maximum cardiac output is developed. There have been too few measurements of this value in Olympic-class athletes, but a figure of 30 to 40 liters per minute seems probable for participants in endurance events (Table 2). The maximum pulse rate is no higher in the athletes than in unfit subjects; indeed, it may be a little lower, although the reported differences probably reflect difficulties encountered by athletes in reaching true maxima while performing standard physiological

Table 2.—Results* Obtained for Five Canadian Endurance Athletes and Five Control Subjects†

Age (yr)	Weight (kg, lb)	Sex	Event	Mode of Exercise	$\dot{Q}$ max (liters/min)	f_h (beats/min)	Q (ml)	Cao_2-Cvo_2 (ml/100 ml)	$\dot{V}o_2$ max (ml/kg/min [STPD])
21	70.8, 156	M	Swimming, ≧400 meters	BE	30.4	183	166	15.3	65.8
21	93.2, 205.5	M	Swimming, ≧400 meters	T	37.3	184	203	15.6	62.7
23	68.3, 150.5	M	Field hockey	T	32.2	187	172	15.4	70.7
40	63.5, 140	F	Long distance running	T	28.1	195	144	14.2	63.6
33	68.7, 151.5	M	Long distance running	BE	30.2	170	177	15.9	70
Mean					31.6	184	172	15.3	66.6
29	78.9, 174	M	Control	T	27.5	195	141	14.1	47.4
25	69.8, 154	M	Control	T	24.5	173	141	12.8	47.2
27	63.2, 139.5	M	Control	T	22.7	191	119	12.6	44.6
34	75.3, 166	M	Control	T	28.3	173	164	13.6	52.3
23	76.3, 168	M	Control	T	25.7	187	137	13.6	50.1
Mean					25.7	184	140	13.3	48.3

*Cardiac output ($\dot{Q}$ max), pulse rate (f_h), stroke volume (Q), arteriovenous oxygen difference (Cao_2-Cvo_2), and maximum oxygen intake ($\dot{V}o_2$ max) during maximum exercise on treadmill (T) or bicycle ergometer (BE). STPD signifies standard temperature and pressure, dry.
†From Simmons.[11]

Table 3.—Probable Distribution of Cardiac Output in Maximal Exercise

	Tissue Volume (liters)	Oxygen Consumption (ml/min [STPD*])	Maximum Flow Per Unit Volume (ml/ 100 ml/min)	Total Flow (liters/min)	Resultant Arteriovenous Oxygen Difference (ml/100 ml)
Muscle	28	4,550	87	24.5	18.6
Skin	10	12	60	6	0.2
Other organs	32	138	4.7	1.5	9.2
All organs†	70	4,700	45.7	32	14.7

*Standard temperature and pressure, dry.
†Total or average.

45

tests. Thus, it seems somewhat unrealistic to measure the performance of a swimmer who is accustomed to arm exercise while prone in cold water by testing him seated on a bicycle ergometer in a warm room. The two main differences of the athlete relative to control subjects are (1) a larger stroke volume and (2) a larger arteriovenous oxygen difference. The probable distribution of the athlete's cardiac output during maximum endurance exercise is shown in Table 3.

The maximum likely muscle blood flow is of the order of 100 ml/100 ml/min, and this maximum may not be achieved in the most active muscles because flow is restricted by activity; thus the major part of the muscle bulk of the body must be exercised to achieve the average muscle flow of 87 ml/100 ml/min that seems likely during maximum endurance exercise.

One "'end point" of endurance exercise in the athlete is an acute circulatory failure. This is typically peripheral in type, a response to (1) increasing skin flow, and (2) relaxation of the venous reservoirs as body temperature rises. The face shows a grey cyanosis, and the gait becomes increasingly uncoordinated as cerebral blood flow falls; consciousness also may be dimmed, and visual scotomata may be reported. Furthermore, if the subject stops abruptly, instead of "warming down," the symptoms may be immediately worsened due to loss of the venous pump mechanism of the leg muscles. Since most of the problem is gravitational pooling, full consciousness is rapidly restored when the athlete becomes prone.

Central circulatory failure has been reported in quadruped animals during treadmill running. In man, discomfort in the hepatic region may be a sign of incipient right ventricular failure, and the pulmonary edema occurring at very high altitudes is evidence that left ventricular failure can also occur. However, in general, an athlete who is free of cardiac and respiratory disease seems unable to push himself to the state reflected in that unfavorable part of Starling's curve in which an increase of diastolic volume is associated with a decrease of cardiac output. This may be partly because a smaller fraction of the body musculature is active in man

46

than in a quadruped, and partly because performance in upright subjects is limited by peripheral circulatory factors before the point of central failure is reached.

As in isometric stress, the two commonest causes of death in endurance events seem to be rupture of a previously unsuspected aneurysm, and coronary insufficiency. The increase of systemic blood pressure and of cardiac work load are less intense in endurance than in isometric exercise, but their longer duration leads to at least an equal number of untoward incidents. Burton[5] has suggested that in some cases, harm may result from the increased coronary flow induced by exercise. The pressure drop across any atheromatous plaques in the coronary vessels, is increased, thereby predisposing to hemorrhage into the plaques and total occlusion of the vessels. However, when death is sudden, the usual immediate cause is ventricular fibrillation; in exercise this tends to be triggered not only by patchy hypoxia of the myocardium, but also by the high level of circulating catecholamines.

Repeated endurance exercise gives rise to substantial hypertrophy of the myocardium, and at one time it was believed that the "enlarged heart" of the ex-athlete was a serious embarrassment. However, it is now generally accepted that where an adverse long-term effect on health has been seen, this has been because the ex-athlete finds difficulty in regulating his appetite to a level appropriate for a sedentary life.[12] He becomes obese, and this in turn increases his liability to cardiovascular disease.

Protracted Stress

In protracted exercise, the limiting factors become increasingly the thermoregulatory capacity of the athlete, his ability to maintain an appropriate fluid balance, and the extent and mobility of the available food reserves. Deep body temperatures of 105.8 F (41 C) have been recorded in runners even at low ambient temperatures approximately 68 F,[13] and the demand for skin blood flow is met by further diversion of cardiac output from the viscera.[14] Some protest on the part of the affected tissues is normal; albumin and occasional red blood cells are found in the urine, and the plasma contains increased quantities of enzymes associated with tissue injury. Progress to hyperpyrexia, adrenocortical failure, or renal failure is possible under adverse climatic conditions.

Marathon runners tolerate a 3% to 7% water loss surprisingly well,[15] but it is obviously prudent to supply as much fluid as possible to contestants in the form of glucose and saline solutions; volumes of up to 1 liter per hour are tolerated, but if gastric distension is to be avoided, the concentration of glucose should not exceed 5%. In events such as the marathon, advantage should also be taken of as much tepid sponging as the rules of the contest permit.

Constitutional Factors

Both the average personality and transient variations of mood markedly influence the extent of the psychological stress induced by competition. Habituation to a strange environment is thus an important part of the preparation of an Olympic athlete, irrespective of the altitude of the sports arena.

Body build has an important influence on the work performed, and thus upon the circulatory stress involved in endurance events such as running. For a given pace, the endomorph with his large deposits of fat is at a serious disadvantage, and to the extent that bulk is developed in muscles not needed for a specific contest, the muscular mesomorph is also at some disadvantage relative to the lean and thin ectomorph.

Transient Variations of State

Training will decrease the relative circulatory cost of exercise at a specific pace partly because there is an increase in an individual's maximum cardiac output[9] and partly because the efficiency of performance is improved. However, athletes always perform so close to their maximum capacity that the most important variable is probably their state of training relative to that of their rivals. In general, the athlete who is outclassed runs in a poorly coordinated manner, and is much nearer to circulatory failure than the successful contestant.

Various acute infections may influence the circulatory status adversely. Myocardial infections are an obvious contraindication to participation. Gastrointestinal tract infections may reduce the circulatory blood volume and increase the stress of endurance and protracted events, while the reported episodes of pulmonary edema are commonly linked with a history of acute respiratory infection.

48

Diet is important mainly in that visceral blood flow is increased following ingestion of food and fluids; if food is necessary during protracted exercise, it should be taken in a form that does not impair gastric emptying.

Influence of Environment

Physiological adjustment to altitude change is discussed by another contributor to this issue; however, certain specific influences of the altitude of Mexico City (approximately 7,350 ft) on the circulatory system deserve emphasis. The oxygen content of the arterial blood will be reduced by about 1 ml/100 ml. This will not have much influence on the active muscles, since these are already extracting oxygen fairly completely from the blood stream; however, it may increase the tendency to hypoxia in the viscera and the myocardium, with earlier onset of cerebral hypoxia and peripheral circulatory failure.

Hypoxia also increases the discharge from the aortic and carotid chemoreceptors, and this together with some hypocapnia from overventilation will increase the tendency to hypertension prior to exercise. The recovery phase will also be prolonged by hypoxia, and in this connection it is noteworthy that one of the more frequent complaints of athletes who have competed in Mexico City is stiffness of the muscles eight to ten hours after a contest. This cannot represent a persistent accumulation of lactic acid, since the half-time of oxidation of anaerobic metabolites is approximately 15 minutes. Possibly, hypoxia leads to a greater permeability of the muscle capillaries, with increased exudation of tissue fluid. If so, the stiffness should be remedied by breathing oxygen for a few minutes following a race.

The possibility of inducing "high altitude" pulmonary edema by exercise in Mexico City has also been mooted. There are certain grounds for optimism. There are currently no recorded cases which have occurred at less than 10,000 ft, and at this altitude, the reduction in oxygen content of the arterial blood is at least twice that found in Mexico City. The 1955 Pan-American Games were also held in Mexico without any problem. On the other hand, known cases have followed normal daily work in the mines, and it would be surprising if the energy expenditures of the affected individuals averaged over an eight-hour shift were more than 50% of their aerobic power. There thus seems at least a chance of precipitating pulmonary edema by the maximum efforts of a world contest at 7,350 ft.

Heat has been a problem increasing the circulatory stress in some Olympic contests. However, in Mexico City the altitude gives a dry and relatively cool climate; at the time of the 1968 contests it is likely that the temperature will be 70 to 80 F, without excessive humidity.

Oxidant air pollution has recently attracted attention as a possible factor limiting athletic performance[16]; if substantiated, the possible circulatory or respiratory basis for the loss of performance remains to be determined. However, Mexico City is a densely populated conurbation surrounded by mountains, and has a high intensity of solar radiation. The situation favors air pollution, and while I know of no specific measurements, a substantial oxidant contamination of the atmosphere seems probable.

The energy expenditure and thus the circulatory stress for a given rate of performance will also be affected quite markedly by wind and rain at the track.

Specific Medical Recommendations

The general basis of medical examination for an Olympic contest will naturally follow the format recommended for inclusion in the Olympic Medical Archives (Olympic Museum, Mon Repos, Lousanne, Switzerland), but a few specific points may be added. First, oxygen transport depends equally upon the cardiac output and the hemoglobin level of the blood.[6] Athletes quite commonly suffer from anemia; this has been blamed on iron loss in sweat, and on an increased destruction of red blood cells by the high rate of blood flow, but could equally be the consequence of a "faddy" diet. Assurance of a normal hemoglobin level, with iron and vitamin supplements taken as necessary, is an important means both of reducing hypoxic stress and of improving performance in Mexico City. Second, some attempt should be made to eliminate from the contests individuals liable to the two commonest causes of accidental circulatory death—aneurysmal rupture and coronary ischemia. Berry aneurysms of the arterial circle of Willis can only be located by the rather drastic procedure of cerebral angiography, but aneurysms and sclerosis of

50

the great vessels can be detected by careful inspection of standard posteroanterior roentgenograms of the chest. Coronary ischemia can readily be evaluated by the simple expedient of recording a chest ECG during maximum exercise in the laboratory; depression of the ST segment should not exceed 0.2 mv, and frequent ventricular extrasystoles or atrioventricular block developing during or immediately following exercise are further warning signs of myocardial ischemia. The hazards of renal failure during prolonged exercise are undoubtedly increased if there is proteinuria or hypertension at rest, and either finding should indicate the need for a complete evaluation of renal function. Finally, the risks of acute myocardial failure and of pulmonary edema are both increased by acute infections, and it would thus seem a wise precaution to keep a daily record of the oral temperature of all contestants when they are at rest.

The work of the laboratory is supported in part by research grants from the Department of National Health and Welfare, Ottawa, and from the Ontario Heart Foundation.

References

1. Åstrand, P.-O.: Concluding Remarks: International Symposium on Physical Activity and Cardiovascular Health, *Canad Med Assoc J* **96**:907-911 (March 25) 1967.

2. Taggart, P., and Fibbons, D.: Motor-Car Driving and the Heart Rate, *Brit Med J* 1:411-412 (Feb 18) 1967.

3. Brod, J., et al: Circulatory Changes Underlying Blood Pressure Elevation During Acute Emotional Stress (Mental Arithmetic) in Normotensive and Hypertensive Subjects, *Clin Sci* **18**:269-279 (May) 1959.

4. Bogdonoff, M.D., et al: Cardiovascular Responses in Experimentally Induced Alternations of Affect, *Circulation* **20**:353-359 (Sept) 1959.

5. Burton, A.C.: *Physiology and Biophysics of the Circulation,* Chicago: Year Book Medical Publishers, Inc., 1965.

6. Shephard, R.J.: "An Integrated Approach to Performance at Sea Level and at an Altitude of 7,350 ft," in *Proceedings of Fifth Pan-American Congress on Sports Medicine, Winnipeg, Canada, 1967,* to be published.

7. Kirch, E.: Anatomische Grundlagen der Sportherzens, *Verh Deutsch Ges Inn Med* **47**:73-98, 1935.

8. Johnson, W.R.; Hutton, D.C.; and Hohnson, G.B.: Personal Traits of Some Champion Athletes as Measured by Two Projective Tests, Rorschcah and H.T.P., *Res Quart Amer Assoc Health Phys Educ* **25**:484-488 (Dec) 1954.

9. Lind, A.R., and McNicol, G.W.: Muscular Factors Which Determine the Cardiovascular Responses to Sustained and

Rhythmic Exercise, *Canad Med Assoc J* **96:**706-713 (March 25) 1967.

10. Jokl, E.: *The Clinical Physiology of Physical Fitness and Rehabilitation,* Springfield, Ill: Charles C Thomas, Publisher, 1958.

11. Simmons, R.E.: *Effect of Physical Conditioning Upon the Cardiovascular Circulation,* thesis, University of Toronto, 1968.

12. Montoye, H.J., et al: The Longevity and Morbidity of College Athletes, *Phi Epsilon Kappa* Fraternity, USA, 1957.

13. Bazett, H.C.: "The Regulation of Body Temperature," in Newburg, L.H. (ed): *Physiology of Heat Regulation and the Science of Clothing,* Philadelphia: W. B. Saunders Co., 1949.

14. Rowell, L.B., et al: "Effects of Strenuous Exercise and Heat Stress on Estimated Hepatic Blood Flow in Normal Men," in Karvonen, M.J., and Barry, A.J. (eds.): *Physical Activity and the Heart,* Springfield, Ill: Charles C Thomas, Publisher, 1967.

15. Saltin, B.: "Body Temperature and Sweating During Severe Exercise," in *Proceedings of the Fifth Pan-American Congress on Sports Medicine, Winnipeg, Canada, 1967,* to be published.

16. Wayne, W.S.; Wehrle, P.F.; and Carroll, R.E.: Oxidant Air Pollution and Athletic Performance, *JAMA* **199:**901-904 (March 20) 1967.

THE ELECTROCARDIOGRAMS OF DAILY RUNNERS

W.P. Leary, M.Sc., M.B. (Rand), F.C.P. (S.A.), M.R.C.P. (Lond.),
and J.K. McKechnie, B.Sc. Hons., M.D. (Rand), M.R.C.P. (Edin.)

Most medical practitioners are aware that the death rate from ischaemic heart disease has risen sharply in recent years. Ryle and Russell[1] have pointed out that Osler was admitted F.R.C.P. before seeing a single case of angina pectoris, whereas most clinical students are acquainted with the condition today. Campbell[2] has suggested that this state of affairs is largely due to the increasing age of the general population and that changes in environment are probably of little importance.

Master and Rosenfeld,[3] Brody,[4] and Rumball and Acheson[5] are among those who have established that cardiographic evidence of myocardial ischaemia after exercise tests identifies individuals with a high risk of future overt coronary artery disease. Since Currens and White,[6] Brunner[7] and Raab[8] have expressed the opinion that regular exercise is of some value in preventing myocardial infarction, we thought it pertinent to present our preliminary findings in a group of daily runners in whom unequivocal evidence of ischaemic heart disease, as judged by postexercise electrocardiograms, is lacking.

SUBJECTS AND METHODS

Thirty-five men belonging to a Durban club were examined. Most are business or professional men and meet during lunch-break for their daily run on a city field. Small groups run at varying speeds and for distances of 2 - 10 miles, depending upon inclination and available time. No attempt was made to grade the men in terms of athletic ability or daily mileage, but all those included in the study were between 28 and 64 years of age and had been running regularly for at least a year when the tests were carried out.

TABLE I. PRE-EXERCISE

Subject	Age	Rate	A°QRS	P – R	QRS	R – R	Q – T	Q – Tc	Remarks
1	65	—	+50	—	—	—	—	—	S₂, S₃ pattern anti-clockwise rotation
2	46	90	+55	0·14	0·08	0·69	0·34	0·40	
3	33	55	+60	0·14	0·08	1·08	0·40	0·40	
4	46	55	+60	0·18	0·08	1·10	0·40	0·38	
5	48	52	-45	0·20	0·12	1·16	0·40	0·37	
6	41	63	-15	0·20	0·08	0·96	0·36	0·36	
7	29	58	+100	0·18	0·08	1·04	0·40	0·39	
8	60	59	+60	0·16	0·08	1·02	0·46	0·45	
9	39	80	+40	0·18	0·08	0·74	0·38	0·44	
10	40	60	+35	0·16	0·08	1·01	0·38	0·38	
11	43	44	+40	0·18	0·08	1·34	0·44	0·38	
12	46	95	+78	0·14	0·10	0·60	0·32	0·41	
13	38	—	—	—	—	—	—	—	
14	42	69	+60	0·14	0·10	0·88	0·40	0·42	
15	33	—	—	—	—	—	—	—	T waves inverted in III and AVF
16	46	57	+60	0·14	0·08	1·05	0·44	0·43	
17	35	—	—	—	—	—	—	—	
18	40	95	+30	0·16	0·09	0·60	0·32	0·41	T inverted in III and AVF, T flat in V₆
19	35	—	—	—	—	—	—	—	
20	47	66	+60	0·12	0·08	0·92	0·41	0·42	
21	35	75	+90	0·16	0·07	0·80	0·33	0·37	
22	48	85	+60	0·18	0·09	0·72	0·42	0·49	
23	41	60	+80	0·20	0·08	1·00	0·38	0·38	
24	43	52	-15	0·18	0·08	1·16	0·40	0·37	
25	38	80	+80	0·18	0·07	0·73	0·32	0·38	
26	59	46	+60	0·13	0·08	1·32	0·42	0·36	T biphasic and inverted in III and AVF
27	32	54	+30	0·18	0·08	1·18	0·24	0·22	
28	32	50	+75	0·18	0·09	1·30	0·42	0·37	
29	45	62	+75	0·18	0·08	1·02	0·36	0·35	
30	32	54	+50	0·18	0·07	1·06	0·40	0·39	
31	40	65	+75	0·18	0·09	1·00	0·40	0·40	
32	37	45	+45	0·14	0·08	1·32	0·42	0·37	
33	30	55	+100	0·22	0·09	1·10	0·36	0·34	
34	29	58	+62	0·24	0·04	1·04	0·38	0·37	
35	28	58	+84	0·16	0·08	1·00	0·26	0·26	
Mean	40·6	63	+52	0·165	0·08	0·97	0·37	0·37	

Each subject was asked to run a minimum distance of 600 yards at a speed which would induce severe breathlessness, such that he was forced to stop. An electrocardiograph was set up in the pavilion beside the field and tracings were made immediately after the run and at intervals of 2, 4 and 6 minutes. In 19 cases the shorter run was not used and cardiograms were recorded immediately after a marathon. These results have already been reported elsewhere.[9] In 5 cases no control recording could be obtained.

RESULTS

The results of this study are set out in Tables I and II. The mean electrical axis was $+52°$ before and $+57°$ after exercise. This difference is not significant. In none of the subjects examined did the axis shift to the left, and in only 5 of the 30 subjects was there an axis shift to the right of more than $10°$. This right-axis shift was reported by Kahn and Simonson[10] as a feature of a normal effort response.

Runners 1 and 5 had tall P waves in lead II suggesting right atrial pressure increase. Three men had definite T wave inversion in leads III and AVF. This change was present both at rest and after exercise. In runner 16 inversion was more marked at rest than after exertion.

The mean Q-Tc was 0·37 before effort and 0·41 after effort. These values do not represent any significant feature, as the Q-Tc value has limitations,[11] and none of the equations which relate the resting Q-T interval to heart rate is applicable to the tachycardia of exercise. The adaptation of the Q-T interval to the heart rate is a slow process, but an increase in Q-Tc of 0·04 for an increase of mean heart rate from 56 to 90 beats per minute has been recorded in normal subjects.[11]

The mean P-R interval was 0·165 seconds before and 0·16 seconds after exercise. This is not unexpected seeing that the P-R value remains within the normal limits at rates between 60 and 115 beats per minute.[11]

One subject had occasional ventricular extrasystoles after exercise. Another subject whose electrocardiogram had shown a partial heart block of the Wenckebach type during a previous investigation was normal on this occasion, both before and after exercise. None of the subjects examined had any evidence of S-T segment depression.

DISCUSSION

White[12] has stated that the ECG may be normal in 25% of patients with angina pectoris and, because of the difficulty in diagnosing abnormality, stress tests have been conducted to increase the diagnostic sensitivity of ECGs. Positive tests are usually indicative of latent coronary insufficiency, but varying types of stress may be used, and the information derived from these is additive.

TABLE II. FOUR MINUTES AFTER EXERCISE

Subject	Age	Rate	A°QRS	P – R	QRS	R – R	Q – T	Q – Tc	Remarks
1	65	84	+80	0·14	0·10	0·74	0·38	0·44	RSr_1S_1 noted in V1, P 3 mm. peaked in II
2	46	100	+60	0·18	0·10	0·59	0·34	0·44	
3	33	78	+55	0·12	0·08	0·74	0·36	0·41	
4	46	65	+66	0·16	0·09	0·94	0·38	0·39	S_2, S_3 pattern, P 3 mm. peaked
5	48	94	−60	0·16	0·10	0·62	0·30	0·39	
6	41	72	−8	0·18	0·08	0·84	0·36	0·39	
7	29	71	+100	0·18	0·08	0·84	0·32	0·35	
8	60	120	+70	0·16	0·08	0·86	0·36	0·38	
9	39	86	+40	0·16	0·08	0·68	0·30	0·36	
10	40	65	+30	0·16	0·08	0·72	0·34	0·40	
11	43	95	+40	0·16	0·10	0·92	0·40	0·42	
12	46	100	+80	0·14	0·10	0·60	0·32	0·41	
13	38	90	+45	0·16	0·07	0·60	0·32	0·41	
14	42	100	+55	0·14	0·08	0·68	0·38	0·45	
15	33	90	+75	0·16	0·08	0·60	0·38	0·46	
16	46	80	+58	0·14	0·08	0·68	0·34	0·40	T waves flat in III and AVF
17	35	142	+80	0·18	0·08	0·80	0·40	0·45	
18	40	90	+22	0·12	0·08	0·42	0·32	0·49	
19	35	86	+60	0·14	0·08	0·68	0·32	0·38	
20	47	85	+60	0·12	0·08	0·72	0·36	0·42	
21	35	88	+90	0·16	0·08	0·72	0·32	0·37	T inverted in III and AVF
22	48	94	+65	0·14	0·08	0·66	0·32	0·39	
23	41	87	+90	0·16	0·07	0·62	0·30	0·39	
24	43	118	−15	0·12	0·08	0·70	0·36	0·42	
25	38	72	+80	0·20	0·06	0·53	0·32	0·43	
26	59	100	+60	0·15	0·10	0·84	0·36	0·39	Premature ventricular beats
27	32	100	+30	0·18	0·08	0·60	0·36	0·46	
28	32	100	+75	0·16	0·09	0·60	0·32	0·42	
29	45	96	+75	0·18	0·08	0·68	0·32	0·42	
30	32	94	+75	0·16	0·08	0·68	0·30	0·38	T inverted in III and AVF
31	40	94	+45	0·16	0·08	0·64	0·33	0·36	
32	37	100	+100	0·12	0·09	0·60	0·30	0·41	
33	30	72	+62	0·20	0·04	0·86	0·32	0·39	
34	29	72	+86	0·18	0·08	0·86	0·34	0·34	
35	28	115		0·14	0·08	0·52	0·40	0·56	
Mean	40·6	91	+57	0·16	0·08	0·69	0·34	0·41	

Sandberg[13] has stated that the only basis for making a diagnosis of coronary artery disease in an apparently normal individual is the appearance of S-T segment depression of 1·0 mm. or more after maximal exercise. Robb et al.[14] have shown that the death rate from coronary heart disease is 10 times greater in persons who have depression of the S-T segment greater than 0·5 mm. after exercise than in persons with no such change or isolated T wave changes only. In Brody's study[4] and in the study of 660 apparently healthy men by Rumball and Acheson[5] similar findings have been reported.

None of the cardiograms examined in this group of daily runners shows S-T segment depression either before or after exercise. This is in marked contrast with the findings of Doan et al.,[15] Brody,[4] Robb et al.[14] and Rumball and Acheson[5] in their studies of the general population. Indeed, Doan et al. found evidence of ischaemic heart disease in 28% of subjects aged 50 - 54 years. Three of the runners in this series had T wave depression in leads III and AVF, and it should be stressed that these changes were apparently not induced by exercise. Many authorities would regard such changes as being non-specific; T wave inversion induced by effort is however of great significance. Brody[4] found that only 3·6% of his patients with initial T wave abnormalities subsequently developed overt ischaemic heart disease.

Before this investigation one 29-year-old man was known to have a partial heart block of the Wenckebach type. This disappeared during exercise and 14 days after stopping his daily run the resting electrocardiogram also reverted to normal. He began running again and when tested on this occasion—6 months after the 14-day rest period—had a P-R interval of 0·24 seconds at rest with a heart rate of 58 beats/min. There is no clinical evidence of heart disease and this subject, a medical practitioner, can run a mile in about 4 minutes 15 seconds. In 1964 Cullen and Collin[16] reported a similar phenomenon in 2 daily runners, and Manning and Sears[17] have shown that first-degree heart block is not necessarily indicative of organic heart disease but can be a manifestation of increased vagal tone. It seems possible that Wenckebach's arrhythmia has a similar basis in daily runners.

It may be argued that the absence of any electrocardiographic evidence of ischaemic heart disease in a group of men who are asymptomatic and able to run several miles each day is unremarkable or, simply stated, that the results are normal because normal people can run. It is of some interest to note that at least 8 of these men began to take a daily run after the age of 35 years and we think it likely that further investigations carried out on this group of men in the next 10 years will provide further evidence of the value, or otherwise, of regular moderate exercise during the middle years of life.[18]

SUMMARY

The electrocardiograms of a group of 35 men who do daily running have been studied. No evidence of ischaemic heart disease was found.

We wish to thank the Nuffield Foundation and the CSIR, Pretoria, for financial support; Dr D. Bristow of Oregon, USA, for helpful advice; and Mrs Pickthall for assistance in preparing the manuscript.

REFERENCES

1. Ryle, J. A. and Russell, W. T. (1949): Brit. Heart J., **11**, 370.
2. Campbell, M. (1963): Brit. Med. J., **2**, 712.
3. Master, A. M. and Rosenfeld, I. (1961): J. Amer. Med. Assoc., **178**, 283.
4. Brody, A. J. (1959): *Ibid.*, **171**, 1195.
5. Rumball, A. and Acheson, E. D. (1963): Brit. Med. J., **1**, 423.
6. Currens, J. H. and White, P. D. (1961): New Engl. J Med., **265**, 988.
7. Brunner, D. (1961): Circulation, **24**, 896.
8. Raab, W. (1958): Arch. Intern. Med., **101**, 194.
9. McKechnie, J. K., Leary, W. P. and Joubert, S. M. (1967): S. Afr. Med. J., **41**, 722.
10. Kahn, K. A. and Simonson, E. (1957): Circulat. Res., **5**, 629.
11. Simonson, E. (1961): *Differentiation between Normal and Abnormal in Electrocardiography*, p. 158. St Louis: C. V. Mosby.
12. White, P. D. (1930): *Heart Disease*, 2nd ed. New York: MacMillan.
13. Sandberg, L. (1961): Acta med scand., **169**, suppl. 365.
14. Robb, G. P., Marks. H. H. and Mattingly, T. W. (1956): Trans. Assoc. Life Insur. Med. Dir. Amer., **40**, 52.
15. Doan, A. E., Peterson, D. R., Blackman, J. R. and Bruce, R. A. (1965): Amer. Heart J., **69**, 11.
16. Cullen, K. J. and Collin, R. (1964): Lancet, **2**, 729.
17. Manning, G. W. and Sears. G. A. (1962): Amer. J. Cardiol., **9**, 558.
18. Wyndham, C. H. (1969): S. Afr. Med. J., **43**, 720.

Strenuous Exercise Electrocardiogram of Top Class Swimmers in Mexico City

Kizuku Kuramoto, M.D., Michio Ikai, M.D., Kazuo Asahina, M.D.,
Yoshio Kuroda, M.D., Shinkichi Ogawa, M.D., and
Mitsumasa Miyashita, M.Ed.

On 8 top class swimmers electrocardiographic response to the strenuous exercise (60 knee bends in 1 min.) during Mexico training (altitude
2,240 M.) was compared with the response in Tokyo. The increase in
heart rate, relative QT duration, amplitude of P waves, and decrease in
amplitude of T waves with junctional depression of the ST segment were
observed after the exercise. These responses became prominent during
Mexico training both before and after the exercise, and returned to the
previous level after return to Tokyo indicating the effect of the altitude
on the exercise electrocardiogram.

IN Mexico City, where the 1968 Olympic Games is to be held, the partial
pressure of oxygen is about three fourth of the sea level on account of the
altitude of 2,240 M. This report is concerned with the attempt to evaluate
the effect of strenuous exercise in athletes on the electrocardiogram together
with the adaptation to this medium altitude.

Electrocardiographic changes in higher altitude have been found to
reveal right axis deviation, increased terminal QRS vector, right ventricular
hypertrophy and strain.[1]−[6] Various strenuous exercise tests are known to
be sensitive in detecting the minimum coronary insufficiency.[7]−[9] However,
the cardiovascular effect of strenuous exercise at the medium altitude has not
been well defined. In the present study comparisons were made on the
strenuous exercise electrocardiogram during the training in Mexico City
with that of the control study in Tokyo.

MATERIALS AND METHODS

Eight top class swimmers of male with ages between 15 and 26 years (average
22 years) were the subjects of this study. Physical examinations, chest X-ray, resting

The study was supported by the Japanese Sports Association and Japan Amateur Swimming
Federation under the scientific research program for the Mexico Olympic Games.

12 lead electrocardiogram, hemogram and pulmonary function tests were within normal limits in all subjects.

The exercise consisted of knee bends at the rate of 1 bend per sec. for 1 min. ; 60 complete flexions and extensions of the knee and hip joints for 1 min. The routine 12 lead electrocardiogram was recorded before the exercise. Postexercise electrocardiograms were recorded immediately and 2 and 5 min. after the cessation of the exercise in leads I, II, III, V_1, V_4, and V_5.

The control examination was performed during the training in Tokyo (altitude 29 M.) in the middle of September, 1965. During the training in Mexico City (from Sept. 25, 1965 to Oct. 17, 1965), the same examination was performed on every third or fourth day, starting at the second day (Sept. 26) and ending after the competition (Oct. 16). The post-Mexico training examination was carried out on the next day and 3 weeks later after returning to Tokyo (Oct. 21 and Nov. 8).

Serial changes in heart rate, amplitude of P in lead II, mean electrical axis of P and QRS in frontal plane, amplitude of T in lead II, deviation of ST junction in V_5 and relative QT duration[10] before and after the exercise were analysed before, during and after the training in Mexico City.

RESULTS

The average values and the standard deviations of heart rate, amplitude of P and T waves in lead II, and relative QT duration in 8 subjects are shown in Table I. Representative tracings are shown in Fig. 1.

Heart Rate

In control examination in Tokyo the heart rate increased from an average of 56 to 109 beats per min. immediately after the exercise, then decreased to 74 and 65, 2 and 5 min. after the exercise respectively. On the second day in Mexico City the heart rate immediately after the exercise increased to 123 per min., but the heart rates 2 and 5 min. after the exercise were the same as in control examination.

Heart rate during the stay in Mexico City at each timing of exercise is shown in Fig. 2. Resting heart rate increased gradually from 56 to 61 (66 during the competition). Heart rate immediately after the exercise was highest on the second day, and decreased gradually to 119–117, remaining at the higher level than the control value. Heart rate returned to the previous level after coming back to Tokyo.

In 2 cases phasic changes of heart rate showing marked bradycardia was observed 2 min. after the exercise. Occasional ventricular extrasystole appeared immediately after the exercise in 3 cases.

Amplitude of P_{II}

Average amplitude of P_{II} in control examination increased from 1.21 to 1.76 mm. immediately after the exercise, then decreased gradually to 1.50 and 1.32 mm. 2 and 5 min. after the exercise respectively. P_{II} amplitudes

Table I. The Average and Standard Deviation of Electrocardiographic Changes before and after Strenuous Exercise in 8 Swimmers

Days in Mexico					2	5	8	12	16	22		
Date				Sept. 14	26	29	Oct. 2	6	10	16	21	Nov. 8
Heart Rate	Before Exercise		mean	56.0	57.4	57.1	58.9	61.0	61.0	65.9	54.4	57.4
			S.D.	8.0	5.9	8.8	5.3	10.1	11.9	9.1	8.1	9.1
	After Exercise	0′	mean	109.1	123.2	119.3	118.1	118.9	117.3	125.3	115.9	110.5
			S.D.	11.2	10.2	6.2	5.3	8.2	6.8	10.4	10.5	12.0
		2′	mean	75.2	75.9	74.2	72.5	73.0	72.0	81.6	69.0	75.1
			S.D.	10.3	9.1	5.0	10.3	12.7	10.1	10.1	11.6	11.8
		5′	mean	64.5	65.8	71.4	64.6	67.3	66.8	73.4	64.5	66.8
			S.D.	8.1	11.0	6.2	8.3	9.0	8.6	11.3	9.9	7.9
P_{II} Amplitude	Before Exercise		mean	1.21	1.10	0.89	1.36	1.54	1.68	1.58	1.01	0.90
			S.D.	0.39	0.45	0.44	0.75	0.96	0.74	0.64	0.41	0.29
	After Exercise	0′	mean	1.76	2.23	2.11	2.06	2.01	2.00	2.13	1.73	1.60
			S.D.	0.33	0.80	0.62	0.53	0.53	0.52	0.28	0.40	0.43
		2′	mean	1.50	2.03	1.59	1.58	1.74	1.51	1.71	1.32	1.20
			S.D.	0.28	0.43	0.36	0.46	0.50	0.82	0.43	0.41	0.40
		5′	mean	1.32	1.60	1.46	1.43	1.75	1.58	1.65	1.18	1.09
			S.D.	0.25	0.59	0.33	0.58	0.83	0.81	0.56	0.41	0.36
T_{II} Amplitude	Before Exercise		mean	4.25	2.45	3.93	4.58	3.19	2.75	2.68	2.63	3.38
			S.D.	1.27	1.23	1.26	1.08	1.27	1.29	1.49	1.43	1.44
	After Exercise	0′	mean	2.94	1.78	2.88	2.71	1.85	2.27	1.65	1.94	2.30
			S.D.	0.78	1.47	1.35	1.11	1.12	1.17	1.04	0.70	0.99
		2′	mean	3.66	2.66	4.10	3.86	2.83	2.70	2.68	2.56	2.69
			S.D.	1.10	1.62	1.37	0.67	1.23	1.01	1.75	1.06	1.20
		5′	mean	3.63	2.05	3.08	3.69	2.36	2.16	2.11	2.20	2.65
			S.D.	1.00	1.18	1.09	0.84	0.87	1.05	2.23	1.08	1.43
Relative QT Duration	Before Exercise		mean	102.3	107.8	107.9	111.8	107.9	110.2	108.0	103.6	103.0
			S.D.	7.4	5.7	5.7	5.0	5.1	5.3	3.8	4.0	5.4
	After Exercise	0′	mean	105.6	109.6	107.3	112.0	108.8	110.8	109.0	110.5	109.0
			S.D.	5.4	5.6	6.9	6.1	9.3	3.3	6.9	7.5	9.0
		2′	mean	109.5	112.4	113.4	114.1	111.6	114.4	113.6	109.5	108.3
			S.D.	5.8	7.2	5.6	5.3	6.4	6.9	9.9	7.8	6.6
		5′	mean	107.6	112.3	116.8	115.6	114.0	116.0	113.1	111.5	108.6
			S.D.	5.7	7.1	5.1	7.1	7.0	7.3	6.8	6.9	5.7

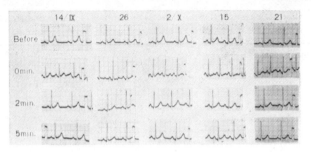

Fig. 1. Representative electrocardiographic response to strenuous exercise before, during and after the Mexico training. T.Y. 26 years old.

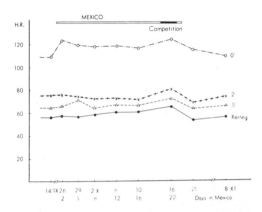

Fig. 2. Changes in heart rate before and after the exercise through Mexico training. 0', 2', and 5' indicate heart rates immediately, 2 and 5 min. after the exercise respectively.

after the exercise were taller during the stay in Mexico City than the corresponding value during the control examination, the most prominent P waves being observed on the second day, giving the average of 2.33, 2.03 and 1.70 mm. immediately, 2 and 5 min. after the exercise respectively. The amplitude of P waves before the exercise increased gradually during the Mexico training; P pulmonale of more than 2.5 mm. was observed in 2 subjects. These P wave changes returned to the previous level on the next day of the return to Tokyo (Fig. 3).

P and QRS axis in frontal plane

Deviation of mean P axis of more than 30° from the control axis was observed in 4 cases, right axis deviation in 3 and left axis deviation in 1. The P axis deviation returned to the previous value after coming back to Tokyo. No QRS axis deviation was observed in the frontal plane throughout the training.

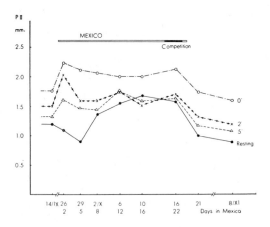

Fig. 3.   Changes in P amplitudes in lead II before and after the exercise through Mexico training.   Symbols are as in Fig. 2.

Amplitude of T in lead II

Amplitudes of T_{II} in control examination were 4.25, 2.94, 3.66, and 3.63 mm. before, immediately after and 2 and 5 min. after the exercise respectively, being lowest immediately after the exercise. T wave 2 min. after the exercise was higher than that of 5 min. after the exercise.   The same pattern of T wave changes was observed during Mexico training.   The amplitude of T waves before and after the exercise decreased on the second day, recovered around a week later, and then decreased again in 12 days of Mexico training. The recovery of the T amplitude to the control level took more than 3 weeks after returning to Tokyo (Fig. 4).

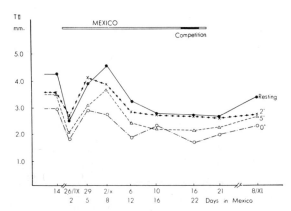

Fig. 4.   Changes in T amplitudes in lead II before and after the exercise through Mexico training.   Symbols are as in Fig. 2.

63

Table II. Number of Cases Revealing ST_J Depression in V_5 among 8 Swimmers

		Days in Mexico			2	5	8	12	16	22		
		ST Depression (mm.)	Date	Sept. 14	26	29	Oct. 2	6	10	16	21	Nov. 8
After Exercise	0 min.	0.5≤	<1.0	2	4	1	4	1	1	0	1	2
			1.0≤	0	1	0	0	0	0	0	0	1
	2 min.	0.5≤	<1.0	2	1	1	2	1	1	1	0	2
			1.0≤	0	2	1	0	1	0	0	0	1
	5 min.	0.5≤	<1.0	0	2	0	0	0	0	0	0	0
			1.0≤	0	0	0	0	0	0	0	0	0

ST junction

No depression of the ST segment or ST junction was observed before the exercise through the training period. Two subjects revealed ST_J depression of more than 0.5 mm. immediately and 2 min. after the exercise in the control study. The ST_J depression after the exercise became remarkable in 5 subjects in the first week of Mexico training, and gradually disappeared in the following days (Table II). The ST depression observed was of the junctional type showing upward ST segment in all cases.

Relative QT duration

Relative QT duration increased after the exercise in all subjects. Average value of the relative QT duration in the control study increased from 102.3% to 105.6%, 109.5% and 108.4% immediately after, and 2 and 5 min. after the exercise respectively. Remarkable increase in relative QT duration at 2 and 5 min. after the exercise was observed throughout the examination.

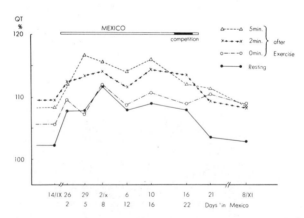

Fig. 5. Changes in relative QT duration before and after the exercise through Mexico training. Symbols are as in Fig. 2.

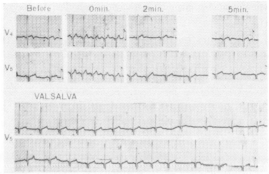

Fig. 6. Marked respiratory variations in R and S amplitudes in V_5 and V_4. Inverted T wave in V_4 became positive after the exercise. Valsalva test also altered the QRS complex.

Relative QT duration both before and after the exercise increased during the Mexico training and returned quickly to the control value after coming back to Tokyo (Fig. 5).

QRS changes

Marked respiratory variations in QRS amplitude immediately after exercise were observed in leads V_4 and V_5, showing decrease in R and increase in S amplitudes during inspiration (Fig. 6). Neither an increase in amplitude of R_{V_1} nor right bundle branch block pattern was recorded throughout the training.

DISCUSSION

The electrocardiographic response to the strenuous exercise of the present examination consisted of the increase in heart rate, relative QT duration, amplitude of P waves, and decrease in amplitude of T waves with junctional depression of the ST segment. These changes became prominent during the Mexico training as compared with the control study in Tokyo. Although it is conceivable that the augmented response in Mexico City may be partly due to the scheduled training, the fact that the same schedule of training was carried out in Tokyo, and the return of these changes to the previous level after coming back to Tokyo may indicate the effect of the altitude on the electrocardiographic response.

The increase in heart rate is the primary factor to increase the cardiac output during and after the exercise,[11] and hypoxia at altitude augmented the response.[12]−[16] The heart rate after the exercise was highest on the second day in Mexico City, followed by a gradual decrease to the new level which is higher than the control level. This may indicate the cardiovascular adaptation to the altitude accompanied with the increase in hemoglobin[17] and respiratory acclimatization.[18]

The relative QT duration in the present study increased 2 and 5 min. after the exercise. The increase in the relative QT duration during the Mexico training may also be a response to the increase in cardiac output. Bruce et al.[19] and Yu et al.[20] observed 7% increase in corrected QT interval or K $(QT/\sqrt{CL})$ during exercise, followed by 9% decrease in the recovery phase. The different response of the relative QT duration to the exercise might be derived from the difference in the grade and duration of the exercise.

Increased amplitude in P waves after the exercise indicated the right atrial overloading due to the increase in cardiac output and sympathetic tone.[8],[21]−[23] The increase in P amplitude after the exercise in Mexico City might be caused by the tachycardia. However, it was observed 2 and 5 min. after the exercise when heart rate revealed little difference from the control examination. During the Mexico training P waves before and after the exercise became peaked, showing P pulmonale at rest in 2 cases, and right axis deviation of P waves was observed in 3 cases. These changes indicated the increased right atrial strain probably from the increased cardiac output and pulmonary vascular resistance at high altitude.[24]

No right ventricular strain pattern such as right ventricular hypertrophy or right bundle branch block was observed in the present study, suggesting the adaptability of the right ventricle to the volume overload.

Decreased amplitude of T waves immediately after the exercise might indicate the extracardiac effect of deep respiration.[25] However, respiratory changes in QRS amplitude was relatively small in lead II, and flattened T waves after the exercise may indicate either an increased sympathetic tone,[8],[26] or an effect of tachycardia on the myocardium.[22] T wave amplitudes 2 min. after the exercise were higher than the T waves 5 min. after the exercise. This may indicate the relative preponderance of vagal tone 2 min. after the exercise. The phasic appearance of bradycardia at this time may also support this interpretation.

Rumball and Acheson[9] observed the junctional ST depression of 1 mm. or more after strenuous exercise in 50% of normal subjects. Wood et al.[27] and Bellet et al.[8] considered the ST_J depression as a normal response. However, the increased prevalence and extent of junctional ST depression after the exercise may suggest a slight myocardial ischemia in the first week of Mexico training. Disappearance of ST depression in the following days may indicate the adaptation to the altitude. Moreover, most of the subjects complained anginal chest pain during and after the race on the competition.

These facts indicated the need for the complete cardiovascular evaluation of the athletes as well as the controlled schedule for the adaptation to this medium altitude.

Summary

The effect of strenuous exercise (60 knee bends in 1 min.) on the electrocardiogram was studied in 8 top class swimmers in Mexico City (altitude 2,240 M.). The electrocardiographic changes during the 3 week Mexico training were compared with the responses in Tokyo.

(1) Heart rate immediately after the exercise increased markedly on the second day in Mexico, and declined gradually. Heart rate before and immediately after the exercise remained at higher level during Mexico training than in Tokyo.

(2) Average amplitudes of P waves before and after the exercise in lead II were taller during Mexico training than in control study in Tokyo, the most prominent P waves after the exercise being observed on the second day in Mexico. P pulmonale at rest was observed in 2 cases. Right axis deviation of P waves was observed in 3 cases. These changes in heart rate and P waves returned to the control value after coming back to Tokyo.

(3) Amplitude of T waves in lead II decreased immediately after the exercise throughout the study. Decreased amplitude of T waves before and after the exercise was remarkable after 12 days of Mexico training.

(4) The junctional depression of ST segment after the exercise was remarkable in the first week of Mexico training, and disappeared gradually in the following week.

(5) Relative QT duration was increased 2 and 5 min. after the exercise. Relative QT duration increased during the Mexico training both before and after the exercise.

These electrocardiographic changes during Mexico training and anginal chest pain experienced during and after the race indicated the need for the careful health examination of the athletes.

References

1. Penñaloza, P., Gamboa, R., Dyer, J., Echevarria, M., and Marticorena, E.: Am. Heart J. **59**: 111, 1960.
2. Peñaloza, P., Gamboa, R., Marticorena, E., Echevarria, M., Dyer, J., and Guitierrez, E.: Am. Heart J. **61**: 101, 1961.
3. Rotta, A. and López, A.: Circulation **19**: 719, 1959.
4. Milledge, J. S.: Brit. Heart J. **25**: 291, 1963.

5. Jackson, F. and Davies, H.:   Brit. Heart J. **22**: 671, 1960.
6. Recararren, S. and Arias-Stella, J.:   Brit. Heart J. **26**: 806, 1964.
7. Doan, A. E., Peterson, D. R., Blackmon, J. R., and Bruce, R. A.:   Am. Heart J. **69**: 11, 1965.
8. Bellet, S., Eliakim, M., Deliyiannis, S., and Figallo, E. M.:   Circulation **25**: 686, 1962.
9. Rumball, C. A. and Acheson, E. D.:   Brit. Heart J. **22**: 415, 1960.
10. Lepeschkin, E.:   Modern Electrocardiography, The Williams and Wilkins Co. p. 183, 1951.
11. Rushmer, R. F., Smith, O., and Franklin, D.:   Circulat. Res. **7**:   602, 1959.
12. Theilen, E. O., Gregg, D. E., and Rotto, A.:   Circulation **12**: 383, 1955.
13. Balke, B.:   Am. J. Cardiol. **14**: 796, 1964.
14. Pugh, L. G. C. E.:   J. Appl. Physiol. **19**: 441, 1964.
15. Pugh, L. G. C. E., Gill, M. B., Lahiri, S., Milledge, J. S., Ward, M. P., and West, J. B.:   J. Appl. Physiol. **19**: 431, 1964.
16. Astrand, P. O. and Astrand, I.:   J. Appl. Physiol. **13**: 75, 1958.
17. Pugh, L. G. C. E.:   J. Physiol. **170**: 344, 1964.
18. Schilling, J. A., Harvay, R. B., Becker, E. L., Velasquez, T., Wells, G., and Balke, B.:   J. Appl. Physiol. **8**: 381, 1956.
19. Bruce, R. A., Livejoy, F. W., Pearson, R., Yu, P. N. G., Broshers, G. B., and Velasquez, Z.:   J. Clin. Invest. **28**: 1423, 1949.
20. Yu. P. N. G., Bruce, R. A., Lovejoy, F. W., and Pearson, R.:   J. Clin. Invest. **29**: 279, 1950.
21. Smith, W. G., Cullen, K. J., and Thorburn, I. O.:   Brit. Heart J. **26**: 469, 1964.
22. Scherf. D. and Schaffer, A. I.:   Am. Heart J. **43**: 927, 1952.
23. Beckner, G. L. and Winsor, T.:   Circulation **9**: 835, 1954.
24. Banchero, N., Sime, F., Penaloza, D., Cruz, J., Gamboa, R., and Marticorena, E.:   Circulation **33**: 249, 1966.
25. Wasserburger, R. H., Siebecker, K. L., and Lewis, W.:   Circulation **13**: 850, 1956.
26. Wendkos, M. H.:   Am. Heart J. **28**: 549, 1944.
27. Wood, P., McGregor, M., Magidson, O., and Whittaker, W.:   Brit. Heart J. **12**: 363, 190.

NOTCHING IN THE QRS COMPLEX IN THE ELECTROCARDIOGRAMS OF SPORTSMEN[1]

HERTTA RAUNIO, V.-M. ANTTONEN, P. SAVOLA, and L. PYYKÖNEN.

ABSTRACT

Secondary upright deflection of the QRS complex in the right precordial leads and for significant terminal notches (notches during the terminal 0.04 seconds of the QRS complex) were looked for in the electrocardiograms of 21 top league football players, and in electrocardiograms of 22 champion class skiers. Vectorcardiograms of the 21 football players taken during the competition season were also studied.

A secondary upright deflection in the right precordial leads was found in the electrocardiograms of 17 of the football players and 13 of the skiers, and a significant terminal notch in those of two football players and two skiers.

A terminal appendage pointing to the right and upwards was found in the QRS sÊ loop of 14 football players. Except in one case, the secondary upright deflection in the right precordial leads appeared before the start of the terminal appendage, simultaneously with an anterior displacement of the returning limb of the QRS sÊ loop. This secondary upright deflection of the QRS complex in the right precordial leads is believed to be due to right ventricular preponderance. The deflection was not related to a significant terminal notch.

The electrocardiograms of trained athletes frequently display unusual features in the QRS complex. In 1934 Wilson observed a broad S wave in lead I, associated with an abnormally long QRS duration in the electrocardiograms of athletes (19). Klemola (1951) in a series of athletes, found a widening and notching of the QRS complex of no clinical significance (8). Isaacs et al. (1962) mentions »notching and/or shouldering» in the ascending limb of the S wave in lead V_1, he found it more frequently among wrestlers and weight lifters than among untrained subjects (7). Another pattern frequently seen in the electrocardiograms of athletes is an RSR' pattern, as well as slurring of the S wave in lead V_1 (5, 13, 14, 16, 17). Roskamm et al.

report that the larger the heart, the more frequently did this pattern occur, and it was considered to be a result of hypertrophy and dilatation of the right ventricle (14).

In our previous paper we stated that although a significant terminal notch (a notch during the terminal 0.04 second of the QRS complex) is usually a sign of myocardial damage, it is occasionally found in healthy subjects, for instance in athletes (12).

Despite the large number of electrocardiographic studies on the QRS complex in athletes, only a few include parallel vectorcardiograms (3, 4, 15). We present here the vectorcardiographic and electrocardiographic results for some of the sportsmen.

[1] Acknowledgement: This study was aided by a grant from the Finnish National Board of Sports.

TABLE 1.

Electrocardiographic data on 21 football players.

Shape of QRS complex in leads V_1 and V_{3R}	Number of players	R' wave in lead		Notched S wave in lead		Duration of S wave 0.01 sec. or more in lead		Significant terminal notch
		V_1	V_{3R}	V_1	V_{3R}	I	V_5	
Group 1 Normal rS complex in V_1 and V_{3R}	4	—	—	—	—	1	—	1
Group 2 Secondary upright deflection lower than preceding R wave in V_1 and/or V_{3R}	7	1	3	2	4	4	1	1
Group 3 Secondary upright deflection higher than preceding R wave in V_1 and/or V_{3R}	10	8	10	2	—	10	6	—
Total	21	9	13	4	4	15	7	2

TABLE 2

Electrocardiographic data on 22 skiers.

Shape of QRS complex in leads V_1 and V_{3R}	Number of skiers	R' wave in lead		Notched S wave in lead		Duration of S wave 0.04 sec. or more in lead		Significant terminal notch
		V_1	V_{3R}	V_1	V_{3R}	I	V_5	
Group 1 Normal rS complex in V_1 and V_{3R}	9	—	—	—	—	4	4	1
Group 2 Secondary upright deflection lower than preceding R wave in V_1 and/or V_{3R}	7	1	3	3	4	5	2	—
Group 3 Secondary upright deflection higher than preceding R wave in V_1 and/or V_{3R}	6	3	6	3	—	5	4	1
Total	22	4	9	6	4	14	10	2

METHODS

The series consists of 21 football players — the team that won the 1966 Finnish championship — and 22 champion class skiers. The age of the football players ranged from 18 to 34 years, with a mean age of 23.1 years, and that of the skiers from 19 to 39 years, with a mean age of 24.7 years.

The electrocardiograms were recorded with a standard direct-writing electrocardiograph at a paper speed of 50 mm per second and a frequency response of 0—200 cycles per second. The electrocardiograms of the football players were taken during the competition season. Several electrocardiograms were taken of the skiers before training, and then at monthly intervals during their eight months' training and competition season, and again three months after this season had ended.

Special attention was paid to secondary and/or late upright deflection of the QRS complex in leads V_1 and V_{3R}. An upright deflection following the first negative deflection in these leads was called an »R" wave» if it rose above the iso-electric line. A secondary upright deflection appearing below the iso-electric line was termed »notched S wave» if its duration was 0.02 seconds or more. The placing of the R' and notched S waves during the QRS complex was noted. A notch during the terminal 0.04 second of the QRS complex was noted if it fulfilled the criteria for a significant terminal notch (2).

Vectorcardiograms of the 21 football players were taken during the contest season. They were recorded with an Atlas 4 electrocardiograph equipped with an oscilloscope, manufactured by Atlas-Werke AG, Bremen. The Grishman cube system of electrode placement was used. The loops were photographed with a Nikkorex-F camera. The sagittal loop was viewed from the left. The loops were interrupted so that each segment represented an interval of 0.0025 seconds.

The vectorcardiograms were reviewed for right ventricular hypertrophy on the basis of the most consistent changes, for instance clockwise inscription of the QRS sÊ loop in the horizontal plane. A slight right ventricular hypertrophy was diagnosed on the following criteria: a half area vector of the QRS sÊ loop in a horizontal plane greater than $+15°$, and/or a ratio in excess of $1:1$ between the maximal anterior displacement and the maximal posterior displacement of the QRS sÊ loop in the same plane (9). In addition we watched for a fingerlike appendage in the terminal part of the QRS sÊ loops, and for a possible anterior displacement of the returning limb of the same loops.

The generally accepted signs of left ventricular hypertrophy were noted in the vectorcardiograms of the football players (3).

The x-ray examinations were carried out, where possible, on the same days as the electrocardiograms. A mean cardiac volume of 350 to 400 ml. per square metre of body surface was regarded as normal (1).

RESULTS

Table 1 gives the electrocardiographic data on the 21 football players, divided into three groups.

The electrical position was vertical in 17 cases, semivertical in 2 cases, and intermediate in 2 cases. The duration of the QRS complex varied from 0.09 to 0.11 seconds.

A secondary upright deflection in the right precordial leads was found in the electrocardiograms of 17 football players, and a significant terminal notch in those of two.

Table 2 gives the electrocardiographic data on the 22 skiers, similarly divided into three groups. Of all the electrocardiograms taken for each skier, we only take into account the electrocardiogram with the most significant features.

The electrical position was vertical in 15 cases, semivertical in 4 cases, and intermediate in 3 cases. The duration of the QRS complex was from 0.09 to 0.11 seconds.

A secondary upright deflection in the right precordial leads was found in the electrocardiograms of 13 skiers, and a significant terminal notch in those of two.

Generally speaking, prominent R' waves were frequently found in lead V_{3R} while lead V_1 for the same subjects revealed an R' wave of lesser altitude or a notched S wave, or in some cases a normal rS shape.

The secondary upright deflection in the right precordial leads usually began rather early (from 0.03 to 0.06 seconds after the start of the QRS complex) and in only three of the 30 subjects with the secondary upright deflection did it begin within the terminal 0.04 seconds of the QRS complex. The duration of the deflection ranged from 0.02 to 0.04 seconds, thus it frequently ceased preterminally. In these three cases the electrocardiographic criteria for a significant terminal notch were not fulfilled (2).

Among the skiers, in four cases in group 2 and in five cases in group 3 (see Table 2), the secondary upright deflection, barely visible in the precordial leads before training, increased gradually

71

during the follow-up period. These changes were still apparent in the electrocardiograms taken three months after the end of the competition season. The subjects with a secondary upright deflection in the right precordial leads did not differ from the rest of the group as regards training conditions, fitness, etc.

During the match season the cardiac volumes of the 21 football players ranged from 385 to 480 ml, with a mean of 408.3

ml per square metre of body surface. They exceeded the normal mean relative volume in six cases.

Table 3 shows the cardiac volumes of 14 skiers examined before training and during the competition season. Eleven skiers had large hearts even before training, and during the competition period the heart size of all 14 skiers exceeded the normal mean cardiac volume. Table 3 shows that in every instance the heart size had increased greatly during the training period (a mean increase of 17 per cent). The heart size of all 14 skiers diminished greatly after the competition period, but in 11 cases it nevertheless remained large. The mean cardiac volume for this group was 470.2 ml per square metre of body surface.

Table 4 gives the vectorcardiographic data on the football players. In all but one of the 21 vectorcardiograms the terminal QRS forces pointed to the right and upwards, and in 14 there was a terminal appendage pointing upwards, backwards and to the right. In 15 vectorcardiograms the preterminal part of the QRS sÊ loop was displaced forwards so that a slight bend was formed, coinciding in time with the secondary upright deflection in the electrocardiogram (Fig. 1).

TABLE 3

Cardiac volume (ml per square metre body surface) of 14 skiers.

	Before training	During competition season
M.R.	475	550
J.L.	390	550
V.H.	480	540
E.H.	420	500
V.K.	540	680
E.H.	390	430
P.K.	400	440
V.K.	500	570
P.I.	500	610
K.P.	530	700
T.M.	430	530
T.K.	470	520
K.K.	440	470
A.T.	500	530
Mean	461.8	544.3

TABLE 4

Vectorcardiographic data on 21 football players.

Shape of QRS complex in leads V_1 and V_{3R}	Number of players	Terminal appendage in QRS sÊ loop pointing right, backwards and upwards	Forwards displacement of preterminal part of QRS sÊ loop	Cases meeting criteria for slight right ventricular hypertrophy
Group 1 Normal rS complex in V_1 and V_{3R}	4	2	—	—
Group 2 Secondary upright deflection lower than preceding R wave in V_1 and/or V_{3R}	7	4	6	4
Group 3 Secondary upright deflection higher than preceding R wave in V_1 and/or V_{3R}	10	8	9	6
Total	21	14	15	10

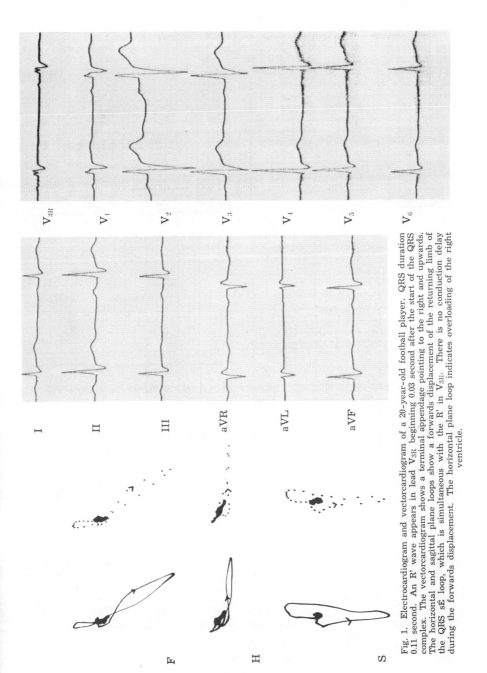

Fig. 1. Electrocardiogram and vectorcardiogram of a 20-year-old football player. QRS duration 0.11 second. An R' wave appears in lead V_{3R} beginning 0.03 second after the start of the QRS complex. The vectorcardiogram shows a terminal appendage pointing to the right and upwards. The horizontal and sagittal plane loops show a forwards displacement of the returning limb of the QRS sE loop, which is simultaneous with the R' in V_{3R}. There is no conduction delay during the forwards displacement. The horizontal plane loop indicates overloading of the right ventricle.

There was no conduction delay during the forwards displacement of the QRS sÊ loop. The inscription of the QRS sÊ loop in the horizontal plane was nowhere clockwise. In two vectorcardiograms a figure 8 was formed in the same plane. In four players in group 2, and in six in group 3, the criteria for slight right ventricular hypertrophy according to Lee and Scherlis were fulfilled (9). Signs of left ventricular hypertrophy were not found in the vectorcardiograms of any of the football players.

DISCUSSION

A secondary upright deflection in the QRS complex in the right precordial leads is frequently associated with a prominent S wave in leads V_5 and V_6 and with a QRS complex duration of 0.07—0.11 seconds. Until recently this R' pattern was called an »incomplete right bundle branch block». A terminal appendage in the QRS sÊ loop pointing to the right and upwards, and usually backwards, has been regarded as a differential-diagnostic sign in vectorcardiograms (10, 11).

Lately, however, investigators have been having second thoughts regarding the »incomplete right bundle branch block». It has been demonstrated that an R' pattern in the right precordial leads may indicate a wide variety of physiological or pathological processes, including right ventricular preponderance (6, 18).

Our present study shows that in the vectorcardiograms of 12 of the football players there was a terminal appendage pointing to the right and upwards with a duration of 0.03—0.04 seconds, while the electrocardiograms of the same subjects showed an R' or notched S wave in the right precordial leads (Table 4).

In all but one case the start of the secondary upright deflection preceded the start of the terminal appendage by 0.02—0.03 seconds. Further, in 15 of the 17 cases with a secondary upright deflection in the electrocardiogram, the returning limb of the QRS sÊ loop was displaced forwards so that a slight bend was formed simultaneously with the

electrocardiographic R' or notched S wave in the right precordial leads (Table 4, Fig. 1).

Our series, therefore, suggests that the secondary upright deflection in leads V_1 and V_{3R} is more probably due to preterminal displacement than to the terminal appendage of the QRS sÊ loop. Thus it appears that an R' wave, though frequently associated with a broad S wave in leads V_5 and V_6, is not of the same origin as an incomplete right bundle branch block pattern.

On the other hand, we found that vectorcardiographic signs of right ventricular hypertrophy are frequently associated with an R' or notched S wave in the electrocardiogram (Table 4).

Here our results agree well with recent findings that cases meeting the formerly accepted electrocardiographic criteria for incomplete right bundle branch block display features associated with right ventricular overload when studied vectorcardiographically (6, 18). Our observation that a secondary upright deflection in V_1 and V_{3R} frequently increases during the training period bears this out.

Possible concomitant hypertrophy of the left ventricle was not considered to be the cause of the secondary upright deflection, especially since vectorcardiographic signs of left ventricular hypertrophy were absent in these subjects.

It should also be noted that the R' or notched S wave pattern had remained unchanged in the skiers three months after their training period had ended. Thus our observation of the persistence of the R' wave agrees with the results of Roskamm et al (14). For this reason we believe that the formation of R' and notched S wave in electrocardiograms of trained athletes is due to a stable myocardial change rather than to a transient condition (e.g. changes in the autonomic nervous system?). It is interesting that 11 of the 13 skiers with a persistent R' or notched S wave still had a large heart after the training and competition period was over. On the other hand, in only six of the 17 football players with a secondary upright deflection in the electrocardiogram did the cardiac volume

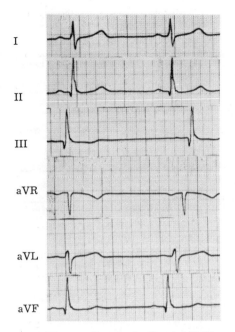
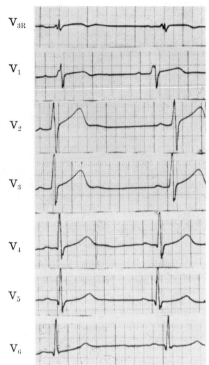

Fig. 2. Electrocardiogram of a 30-year-old skier. Duration of QRS 0.10 seconds. There is a significant terminal notch in the descending limb of the R wave in leads II, III, and aVF. An R' wave is seen in lead V_{3R}. The same formation is found in lead V_1 in the form of a notched R wave. The start of the R' wave precedes the start of the terminal notch by 0.03 second.

exceed the upper limit of the normal mean. The configuration of the heart was normal in these 17 football players. It is well known, however, that a chest x-ray examination is poor at revealing a slight hypertrophy of the right ventricle. Therefore we think it is likely that a secondary upright deflection in the right precordial leads of the electrocardiograms of sportsmen is caused by changes of the myocardium (a preponderance of the right ventricle), poorly seen in x-ray examination.

In our earlier studies a significant terminal notch was only occasionally seen in healthy subjects (2, 12). In the present series four men — two football players and two skiers — had a significant terminal notch (Fig. 2). Two of

them were without the secondary upright deflection in the right precordial leads. In the two remaining cases the R' and notched S waves preceded the start of the significant terminal notch by 0.03 seconds (Fig. 2). In addition, the terminal notches present before training remained unchanged in the electrocardiograms taken during the follow-up period. Thus it is unlikely that the two electrocardiographic patterns mentioned above are of the same origin.

In all of the four electrocardiograms with a significant terminal notch, the notch appeared in one or more of the leads II, III or aVF, placed very low in the descending limb of a tall R wave. These four resemble case 3 — a weight lifter — in our previous paper (12). No clear terminal conduction delay in the QRS sÊ loop was found in any of these vectorcardiograms.

In both of the football players with a significant terminal notch the cardiac volumes during the playing season were 395 and 420 ml per square metre of body surface. In the case of the two skiers, the heart was large (cardiac volume 500 and 680 ml per square metre of body surface) but it diminished after the competition season, so that three months later the cardiac volumes were, respectively, 420 and 540 ml per square metre of body surface, while the terminal notches in the electrocardiograms remained unchanged.

In our earlier study we suggested that, in the presence of pulmonary diseases, the significant terminal notch may be due to hypertrophy of the crista supraventricularis (2). It is possible that in sportsmen, too, the significant terminal notch is caused by a hypertrophied crista supraventricularis.

We conclude that in athletes the secondary upright deflection of the QRS complex in the right precordial leads is due to the right ventricular preponderance frequently found by vectorcardiography. A significant terminal notch, though more frequently seen in athletes than in normal healthy subjects, is not related to this deflection.

REFERENCES

1. *Amundsen P:* The diagnostic value of conventional radiological examination of the heart in adults. Acta Radiol Suppl 181, 1959
2. *Anttonen V-M, Raunio H, Krogerus J, Meurman L:* The significance of a notch during the terminal 0.04 second of the QRS complex in an electrocardiogram. Ann Med Intern Fenn 56: 1, 1967
3. *Arstila M, Koivikko A:* Electrocardiographic and vectorcardiographic signs of left and right ventricular hypertrophy in endurance athletes. J Sport Med 6: 166, 1966
4. *Beswick FW, Jordan RC:* Cardiological observations at the Sixth British Empire and Commonwealth Games. Brit Heart J 23: 113, 1961
5. *Heim E:* The electrocardiogram of long-distance runners (studied in 100 Olympic long-distance ski-runners). Schweiz Z Sportmed 6: 1, 1958
6. *Hirnlowa L, Lukasik S:* The vectorcardiogram in partial right bundle branch block. Kardio Pol 8: 293, 1965
7. *Isaacs MS, Brubaker M, Rasch JPh:* Electrocardiographic »notching» and »shouldering» in athletes and untrained men. Cardiologia (Basel) 41: 121, 1962
8. *Klemola E:* Electrocardiographic observations on 650 Finnish athletes. Ann Med Intern Fenn 40: 121, 1951
9. *Lee Y, Scherlis L:* Some problems in the vectorcardiographic diagnosis of right ventricular hypertrophy. Vectorcardiography 1965. North-Holland Publishing Company, Amsterdam 1966, p. 142
10. *Neri G, Binaghi G, Recalcati P, Spreafico Mazzoleni G, Ruggeri PR:* Il Blocco Focale Destro: Studio Vettorcardiografico. Folia Cardiol 24: 381, 1965
11. *Peñaloza D, Gamboa R, Sime F:* Experimental right bundle branch block in the normal human heart. Amer J Cardiol 8: 767, 1961
12. *Raunio H, Anttonen V-M, Lampainen E, Meurman L:* Terminal QRS force changes in subjects with no heart or pulmonary disease. Ann Med Intern Fenn 56: 159, 1967
13. *Roskamm H, Reindell H, Emmerich J, Schmitz G, Keul J, König K:* Herzvolumen und Leistungsfähigkeit bei einem unvollständigen Rechtsschenkelblock im Ekg. Med Klin 57: 2093, 1962
14. *Roskamm H, Weidenbach J, Reindell H:* Nachuntersuchungen von 18 Sportlern, die vor wenigstens 10 Jahren einen unvollständigen bzw. einen physiologischen Rechtsschenkelblock im Ekg gehabt hatten. Kreislaufforsch 55: 783, 1966
15. *Šanda Z, Král B, Horák J:* Electrocardiographic and vectorcardiographic picture of so-called incomplete block of the right ramus of Tawara in athletes. Cas Lek Cesk 102: 749, 1963
16. *Smith WG, Gullen KJ, Thorburn IO:* Electrocardiograms of Marathon runners in 1962 Commonwealth Games. Brit Heart J 26: 469, 1964
17. *Venerando A, Rulli V:* Frequency, morphology and meaning of the electrocardiographic anomalies found in Olympic Marathon runners and walkers. J Sport Med 4: 135, 1964
18. *Walsh TJ:* Panel discussion on ventricular hypertrophy. Vectorcardiography 1965. North-Holland Publishing Company, Amsterdam 1966, p. 177
19. *Wilson FN:* The significance of electrocardiograms characterized by an abnormally long QRS interval and by broad S-deflection in Lead I. Amer Heart J 9: 459, 1934

TELEMETERED EEG
FROM A FOOTBALL PLAYER IN ACTION[1]

JOHN R. HUGHES AND D. EUGENE HENDRIX

INTRODUCTION

The EEG changes during various types of environmental stress have recently been studied, both in animals (Adey 1963) and in man (Squires *et al.* 1963), especially by telemetry (Sem-Jacobsen 1959; Storm van Leeuwen *et al.* 1963; Walter *et al.* 1966). The present study deals with the EEG changes telemetered from a player engaging in one of the most violent of sporting events[2]. This study was also designed to test the effectiveness of a suspension helmut in safeguarding a player from significant head trauma in the American game of football.

METHODS AND APPARATUS

Electrodes (Type No. EIB, Disc, Grass Instrument Co.) were secured by multiple applications of collodion of a predetermined consistency and were placed on both parietal (P_3 and P_4) and occipital (O_1 and O_2) areas; an electrode at P_z position served as a ground. These electrodes were connected via low-noise Microdot (No. 250-3804) cable (5-6″ in length) to a small ($1\frac{3}{4}″ \times 1\frac{1}{4}″ \times \frac{1}{2}″$) transmitter unit, originally designed for the National Aeronautical and Space Administration. The transmitter unit, powered by a small battery of 6.7 V,

---

[1] Supported by the Riddell, Inc., Chicago, Ill.
[2] For the benefit of non-American readers—American football is quite a different sport from that known under this same name outside the U.S.A. [Editor's note]

77

consisted of two channels of amplification connected to the second stage, the voltage-controlled oscillator (VCO), the output of which was frequency-modulated dependent on the input voltage. The third stage was an adder network and the fourth was the transmitter with an output frequency of 234.2 Mc/sec and a transmission distance of 250–300 yds. The receiver was an FM → Analog Convertor (Genisco Co.), utilizing No. 11 and No. 12 standard IRIG channels, and the recorder was a 2-channel ink-writing transistorized unit (Beckman Instrument Co.). The time constant for the entire system was 0.4 sec.

The football player (W. Campbell), a half-back (offense) of the 1966 Northwestern University team, was prepared with the 5 electrodes by 12:20 p.m. on the day of the game. The electrodes were connected 10 min before the game (12:50 p.m.) to the transmitter, secured within a partition built onto the posterior portion of the helmut. Recordings were taken throughout the afternoon until the end of the game (4:00–4:30 p.m.) without any changes required at the half-time, except for a change to a new battery to insure a voltage over 6.7 V. The antenna and receiving unit were placed in the press box where the investigators were situated. Movies of each play in which the subject was participating were also obtained. Other investigators recorded the amount of impact onto the helmut in the form of g-values of force from tri-axial accelerometers located in the helmut (Reid et al. 1963).

EEG recordings were taken during each of the 10 games of the 1966 football season of Northwestern University. On the day after the game the EEG was analyzed, especially for the dominant frequency of the background rhythm. Although instrumental frequency analysis would have added accuracy to the study, this further complexity would not have significantly changed the results as determined by direct visual inspection with the use of a frequency-ruler.

RESULTS

The EEG was successfully recorded for the duration of most of the games, even under difficult recording conditions, as exemplified in Fig. 1. This figure shows the dominant frequency of the background rhythm as 9.0–9.5 c/sec, usually noted during the portions of the game when the player was resting on the bench. Organized background rhythm usually appeared even while the subject's eyes were open, but occasionally fluctuated in both frequency and amplitude when he was resting on the sidelines, according to the type of action he viewed on the field.

Bench
(End of game - 100°)

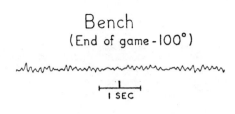

I SEC

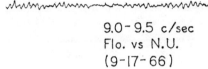

9.0 - 9.5 c/sec
Flo. vs N.U.
(9-17-66)

Fig. 1

Dominant frequency of the background rhythm while the subject was at rest on the bench, but during 100° heat (Florida) on the playing field. In this and remaining figures, top trace is a bipolar recording from the left and the bottom trace from the right parieto-occipital area and calibration shows 50 μV and 1 sec.

Fumble
Impact

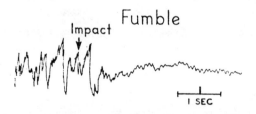

I SEC

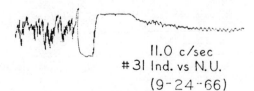

11.0 c/sec
#31 Ind. vs N.U.
(9-24-66)

Fig. 2

The dominant rhythm of 11 c/sec seen after the anxiety of fumbling the ball. Note the muscle and movement artefacts near the time of impact.

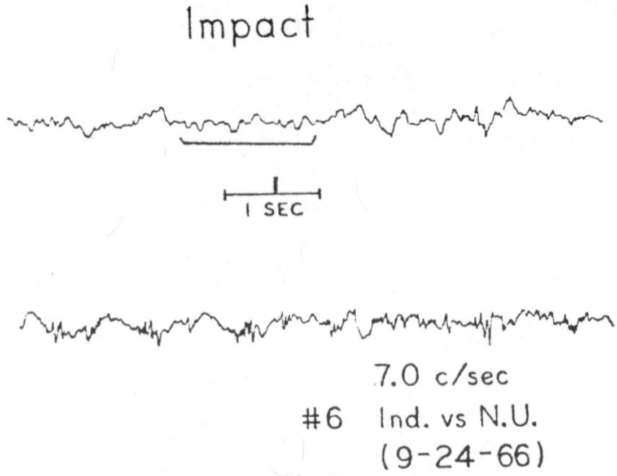

Impact

| SEC

7.0 c/sec

#6 Ind. vs N.U.

(9-24-66)

Fig. 3

Theta rhythms (7 c/sec) seen for a short period of time after severe impact to the head occurring 2 sec before cutout. Note Chan. 1 (above brackets) for the clearer changes of frequency; Chan. 2 includes more muscle and movement artefact.

The greatest variation in the dominant frequency occurred while the subject was playing on the field. Frequencies up to 13 c/sec were often seen during conditions of anxiety and great anticipation. Fig. 2 shows an example of a dominant frequency of 11 c/sec, seen after the subject had fumbled the ball. Other situations in which the dominant frequency was increased above 9.0–9.5 c/sec (resting rhythm) included the anticipation of a kick-off, during the huddle when the next play was indicated, on the line of scrimmage in readiness for the execution of the play, and other conditions like after an (ankle or shoulder) injury and scoring a touchdown. Only rarely were interpretable EEGs recorded during intense action on the field; e.g., while the player carried the ball; however, immediately after the subject was tackled, the EEG was usually interpretable.

The dominant frequency occasionally showed a transitory decrease to theta rhythms, usually after a severe impact to the head (Fig. 3). However, rhythms in the theta range were usually present only for a relatively short period of time (approximately 1 sec), after which the resting rhythm of 9.0–9.5 c/sec was again noted.

Each game was plotted according to the variations in the frequency of the background rhythm. Fig. 4 shows an example of one-half of a game and demonstrates that relatively high frequencies were noted during conditions of anxiety and great anticipation; on two occasions after severe head impact rhythms in the theta range were noted. Usually, just before the beginning of the game a great variation in frequencies was seen, especially during the games considered most crucial by the player.

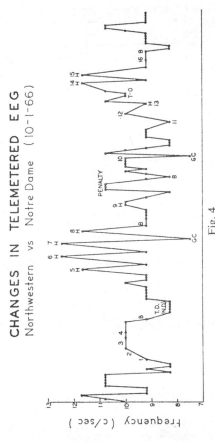

CHANGES IN TELEMETERED EEG
Northwestern vs Notre Dame (10-1-66)

Fig. 4

Variations in the dominant frequency of the background rhythm during the first half of a game. Abscissa: time (approximately 60 min) from near the beginning of the game until the end of the first half. Ordinate: frequency of the dominant rhythm. Numbers indicate the consecutive plays in which the subject was involved. Symbols include: B, on bench; T.D., touchdown; H, huddle; GC, good (head) contact; T-O, time out. Note the variations of frequency just before the first play of the game (No. 1), the high dominant frequency during the huddles (No. 5, 6, 7, 8, 14 and 15), low (theta) frequency after good head contact (No. 7, 10) and the resting rhythm of 9.0–9.5 c/sec during most of the time when the subject was on the bench.

81

DISCUSSION

One of the important points that this study has demonstrated is that the background rhythm is not static, is often present with open eyes and its frequency is constantly changing ("dynamic EEG"). In a routine EEG taken under standard laboratory conditions the frequency of the background rhythm of our subject remained relatively constant during the waking record, contrasting with the frequency changes seen during game conditions.

The rarity of theta waves after head impact and the short duration of this rhythm suggest that our subject did not sustain any significant cerebral trauma. Also, no changes in the resting background rhythm were noted from the beginning to end of the season. Furthermore, after the football season a routine EEG with referential and bipolar recording, 5 min of hyperventilation, photic stimulation, during wakefulness and light sleep failed to show any definite evidence for an abnormality

The relatively high frequencies recorded under conditions of anxiety and great anticipation are consistent with the "hyperexcitability syndrome" (Gastaut 1954). Although Gastaut had referred mainly to the dominant, steady state "resting" rhythms of individuals with certain prominent personality characteristics, it seems reasonable that such rapid alpha rhythms should also appear transiently during periods of great anxiety in individuals who can be generally described as calm and composed. In only very rare instances was a background rhythm of 9.0–9.5 c/sec (the resting rhythm of our subject) recorded when the player was directly involved with the game. Occasionally, when the player sat on the bench, the EEG was fairly accurate in predicting his reactions to the events occurring on the field. The authors are aware that the conclusions in this study are based upon the results of only one subject, but these results seem consistent with known physiological and EEG principles.

It is hoped that this study, involving the successful telemetering of the EEG during one of the most violent of sports, will encourage others in the field to investigate the dynamic aspects of EEG in various life situations.

SUMMARY

1. This study has dealt with the telemetering of the EEG from a football player in action.

2. The dominant frequency of the background rhythm is not static, but is constantly changing ("dynamic EEG") according to the moment to moment changes in the environmental conditions. Relatively high frequencies (up to 13 c/sec) were seen during conditions of great anxiety and anticipation. Rarely, theta rhythms appeared after severe head impact, but their paucity and short

duration suggested that no significant head trauma had occurred.

3. It is hoped that this study will encourage others to investigate the dynamic aspects of EEG in various life situations.

The authors wish to thank W. Campbell, player, Dr. S. Reid, team physician of Northwestern University, originator and coordinator of the project, T. Healion, trainer, and A. Agase, coach, for their aid in making this study possible.

REFERENCES

ADEY, W. R. EEG in simulated stresses of space flight, including vibration and centrifuging. *Electroenceph. clin. Neurophysiol.*, **1963**, *15*: 165.

GASTAUT, H. The brain stem and cerebral electrogenesis in relation to consciousness. In J. F. DELAFRESNAYE (Ed.), *Brain mechanisms and consciousness*. Thomas, Springfield, Ill., **1954**: 249–283.

REID, S. E., TARKINGTON, J. A. and HEALION, T. E. Radio-telemetry in the study of head impacts in football. *Proc. 5th nat. Conf. med. Aspects of Sports*, **1963**: 22–29.

SEM-JACOBSEN, C. W. Electroencephalographic study of pilot stresses in flight. *Aerospace Med.*, **1959**, *30*: 797–801.

SQUIRES, R. D., JENSEN, R. E. and SIPPLE, W. C. Electro-encephalographic changes in human subjects during blackout produced by positive acceleration. *Electroenceph. clin. Neurophysiol.*, **1963**, *15*: 164.

STORM VAN LEEUWEN, W., KAMP, A., KOK, M. L. and ZAAL, J. Monitoring states of alertness by telemetering the EEG. *Electroenceph. clin. Neurophysiol.*, **1963**, *15*: 164.

WALTER, W. G., COOPER, R., CROW, H. J., McCALLUM, W. C., WARREN, W. J., ALDRIDGE, V. S., STORM VAN LEEUWEN, W. and KAMP, A. Contingent negative variation and evoked responses recorded by radio-telemetry in free-ranging subjects. *Electroenceph. clin. Neurophysiol.*, **1966**, *21*: 616.

83

Radio Telemetry of the Electrocardiogram, Fitness Tests, and Oxygen Uptake of Water-Polo Players

A. B. GOODWIN, B.P.E. and

GORDON R. CUMMING, M.D., F.R.C.P.[C]

ELECTRONIC advances have made it possible to transmit various physiologic parameters by means of radio signals and receive these at remote points. One common application of this is the monitoring of heart rate from the telemetered electrocardiogram during various forms of physical activity. The size and weight of the radio transmitters now available permit participation in various athletic events with very little hindrance from the apparatus itself.

The telemetry of heart rate has implications beyond knowledge of heart rate alone. With bicycle exercise, the pulse rate increases in a linear fashion with increases in the intensity of the exercise load, as does the oxygen uptake. This is also true for treadmill exercise.

From the Clinical Investigation Unit of The Children's Hospital of Winnipeg and the Faculty of Medicine, University of Manitoba, Winnipeg.
Supported by the Fitness and Amateur Sport Directorate, Ottawa, Ontario.

Knowing the oxygen uptake *versus* pulse rate relationship from bicycle exercise, it has been postulated that the oxygen demand of a given exercise can be inferred from the pulse rate alone. This postulate assumes that, because pulse rate and oxygen uptake bear a constant relationship to the workload for bicycle or treadmill exercise, the same will hold true for other types of exercise. The present report deals with radio telemetry of heart rate in water-polo players, showing how heart rate can be monitored underwater without special attire; and introduces the problem of pulse rate *versus* oxygen consumption relationships in the swimmer. Maximal and submaximal working capacity tests were also obtained in water-polo participants as a measure of their cardiorespiratory fitness.

Methods

The standard Telemedics radio electrocardiographic transmitter and receiver was used. The bandage-type electrodes supplied with this equipment were not suitable for underwater use. We used silver electrodes 1.0 cm. in diameter, placed in small plastic cups so that the skin-to-electrode contact was entirely dependent on conduction through the electrode jelly. The cups were glued to skin, prepared by scuffing and rubbing with alcohol, with Eastman 910 adhesive. After placing the electrode on the skin, the electrode site was sprayed with a surgical adherent to add to the waterproofing effect of the glued cup electrode itself. No electrode positions will eliminate the muscle artifact of all types of swimming. We have tried four positions: both mid-axillary lines in the sixth interspace; mid-sternum to mid-back; medial end of the right clavicle to the V_5 or V_6 position; and manubrium sterni to xiphisternum. The latter was the best for the majority of swimmers (Fig. 1).

We placed the radio transmitter in a clear plastic box. A plastic or rubber bag would probably be less cumbersome, but the clear box had the advantage of allowing early detection of any leaks. None of the swimmers complained of the added weight or size.

The radio and electrodes were put in place before game time and the player was advised to go out

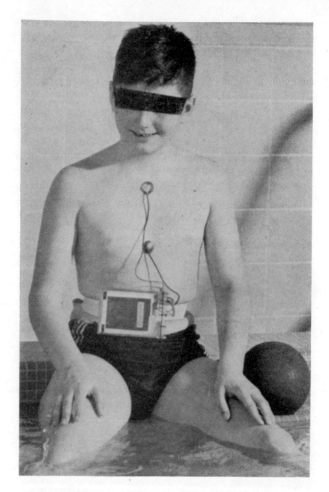

Fig. 1.—Radio transmitter in clear plastic case with belt around waist. Electrodes in position on chest.

and play his normal game. The electrodes were ripped off during the game in two out of eight tests. Electrocardiographic tracings were obtained frequently during the game and at rest periods, and heart rate was obtained by measuring the interval between five beats. No transmitting antenna was required even with the subject totally under-water.

The physical working capacity at a pulse rate of 170 beats/min. (PWC 170) measured in kilopond metres per minute (k.p.m./min.) was determined on an electronically braked bicycle ergometer by methods previously described[1, 2] in 14 water-polo

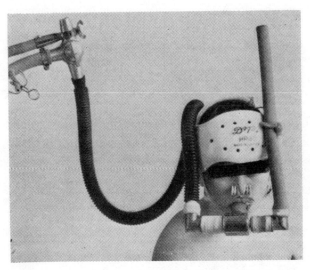

Fig. 2.—Hockey helmet to support air intake and outlet hoses.

players. The workload was then increased to an intensity such that the subject could barely continue the cycling for an additional three minutes. Expired air was collected from the second to the third minute of this maximal exercise for the determination of maximal oxygen uptake. The collected air was analyzed for oxygen using the Beckman paramagnetic oxygen analyzer and for CO_2 using the same instrument.[3] Gas volume was measured with a dry test meter.

Oxygen uptake *versus* pulse rate and workload curves during bicycle exercise was obtained in five of the above subjects on a separate day. Each subject cycled for five minutes at four different loads of increasing severity, and expired air was collected from the fourth to the fifth minute for oxygen uptake measurements. Pulse rates during this study were obtained from an electrocardiogram.

Oxygen uptake was also measured in these five water-polo players by collecting expired air during swimming. A "snorkel" was connected to the intake of a two-way air valve (Fig. 2), the subject's nose

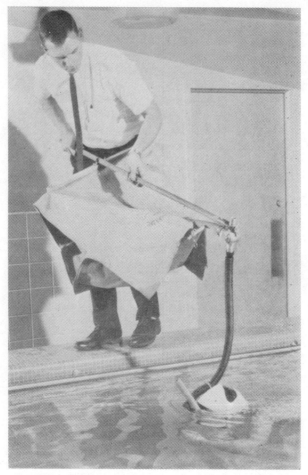

Fig. 3.—Air collection in Douglas bag during swimming.

was clamped, and expired air was collected from the outflow side of the two-way valve in a Douglas bag by going along with the swimmer at pool side (Fig. 3). The swimmer performed at three speeds, slow, medium and near maximum. Pulse rates were monitored during this swimming by the previously described radio technique. The swimmers travelled 50 yards with the mouth piece in and nose clamped before air was collected and 50 yards (or less if unable) for the air collection.

RESULTS

Successful radio telemetric studies were obtained in six of eight players tested during competitive regular league water-polo games. The pulse rates during the various situations of the game are given in Table I. Water polo was played in a 25-yard

TABLE I.—PULSE RATES DURING WATER-POLO GAME

	Pulse rates—beats/min.						
Subjects	1	2	3	4	5	6	Means
Situation:							
1. Resting before game......	127	83	121	117	99	109	109
2. End rest period between periods..............	159	156	175	173	170	—	167
3. Initial sprint to centre....	172	156	167	171	168	188	170
4. Potential score play......	181	188	179	177	183	188	183
5. Offensive ball handling....	179	193	175	181	194	193	186
6. Defensive pursuit........	181	175	170	175	193	191	181
7. Cruising on offence.......	175	192	181	177	194	156	179
8. Cruising on defence......	179	181	170	175	177	181	177
9. Shallow-end pause........	168	166	—	168	170	164	167
10. End of game.............	140	191	179	166	179	—	171
11. Resting rate in laboratory .	66	91	84	84	72	82	80
12. Morning rate at home....	47	71	57	58	48	52	56
13. Maximal rate bicycle ergometer.............	193	194	186	186	183	186	188

pool with a deep and shallow end with four five-minute periods and a two-minute break between periods. No attempt was made to have the player at complete rest just before the game as the anticipative tachycardia from the sport itself, plus an unavoidable excitement from wearing the radio, could not be eliminated.

The maximal pulse rates of 180 to 195/min. were usually obtained during actual scoring or potential scoring plays on offence where the player would be expected to be going all-out, as well as during key defensive plays. The rate during defensive plays tended to be slightly less than for offensive plays, suggesting that most players did not go all-out on defence. However, throughout the entire game, pulse rates remained above 150/min. Even at times of relative inactivity, such as remaining in position in the shallow end resting the feet on the bottom, the pulse rates were over 160/min. At the end of the rest period between periods, pulse rates ranged from 156 to 170 with a mean of 167 beats/min., still far above the pre-game mean of 109 beats/min. Two minutes of recovery was really no better than a slack period in the middle of the game in allowing pulse rate to return towards normal.

It is noted that during the initial sprint to the centre of the pool mean pulse rate increased from

TABLE II.—WORKING CAPACITY AND MAXIMUM OXYGEN UPTAKE OF WATER-POLO PLAYERS

Subject No.	Age (years)	Height (cm.)	Weight (kg.)	PWC 170 (k.p.m./min.)	VO_2 max. l./min.	VO_2 max. ml./kg.	l./min. (standard temp. and pressure) max. vent.	Maximum respiratory quotient	Maximum pulse rate beats/min.
1	25	173	66	1270	3.32	50.0	120.9	1.24	193
2	28	183	82	1230	3.74	45.6	137.4	1.22	194
3	23	180	75	1110	3.47	46.3	126.4	1.22	186
4	19	180	76	1380	4.74	62.4	143.8	1.30	186
5	19	180	75	1422	4.54	60.6	156.3	1.33	183
6	26	183	70	1219	4.04	52.7	136.7	1.33	186
7	26	173	93	1570	4.35	46.7	117.8	1.47	186
8	22	185	95	1365	4.66	49.1	135.8	1.28	190
9	19	180	71	1185	3.82	53.7	146.3	1.25	195
10	35	180	80	1390	4.16	52.0	116.2	1.25	181
11	23	185	69	1322	4.46	64.6	143.1	1.08	195
12	25	178	68	1069	3.50	51.5	136.8	1.32	191
13	37	190	91	1615	4.56	50.2	154.9	1.37	183
14	18	175	61	1191	3.74	60.8	120.1	1.15	196
Mean	25	180	76	1310	4.07	53.3	135.1	1.27	189

109 beats/min. just before to 170 beats/min. in the period of eight to 15 seconds. This rapid mobilization of cardiac reserve is typical of the trained athlete. The mean maximal heart rates for water polo and for bicycle exercise was similar, 186 and 188 beats/min., respectively.

Mean pulse rate immediately after the contest was still above 170 beats/min.

Mean morning minute pulse rate, taken by the subject at home shortly after arising, was 56 (range: 47 to 71), the slow resting rates being in keeping with the above-average fitness of the subjects. Mean resting heart rate in the laboratory after a 20-minute rest was 34 beats/min. greater than the resting rate at home. The mean resting rate just before the start of water polo competition was 29 beats/min. greater than the resting rate in the laboratory and 53 beats/min. greater than the early morning rate at home.

The maximal oxygen uptake and physical working capacity at a pulse rate of 170 of the 14 water-polo players are given in Table II. The maximal oxygen uptake is the best measure of overall fitness available, although there is not complete agreement on how best to express this value. A common method is to give the maximal oxygen uptake in ml./kg. body weight, but the swimmer, who may be more fleshy than the runner, is perhaps unfairly penalized by using weight.

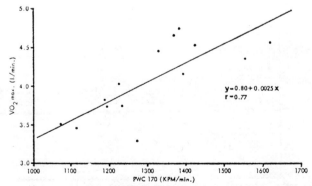

Fig. 4.—Maximum oxygen uptake vs. physical working capacity at a pulse rate of 170 beats/min. (PWC 170). Calculated straight line relationship. Work load is expressed in kilopond metres per minute (k.p.m./min.).

The maximal oxygen uptake of these amateur athletes compares favourably with those of fairly well-trained men in other sports—values of over 50 ml./kg. being quite acceptable. Some of the subjects, particularly those who were a little over-weight, had maximal oxygen uptake values below this figure. Four subjects were above 60 ml./kg. and four were below 50 ml./kg. The two oldest subjects tested (aged 35 and 37 years) both had maximum oxygen uptakes over 50 ml./kg., and both had maximal pulse rates within the same range as the younger subjects.

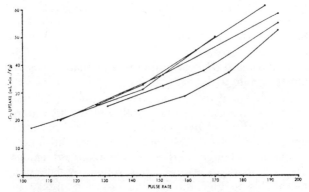

Fig. 5.—Oxygen uptake *vs.* pulse rate for bicycle exercise, five subjects; nearly straight line relationship.

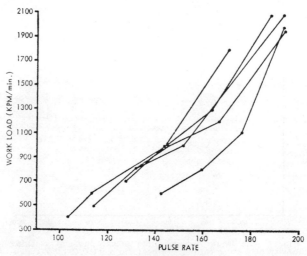

Fig. 6.—Work load *vs.* pulse rate for bicycle exercise, five subjects; nearly straight line relationship.

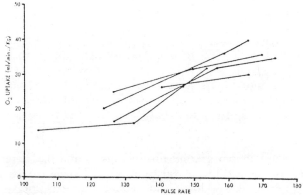

Fig. 7.—Oxygen uptake *vs.* pulse rate for swimming, five subjects.

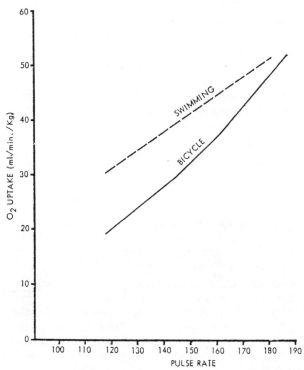

Fig. 8.—Oxygen uptake *vs.* pulse rate for bicycle exercise and swimming—means from five subjects. There is a greater oxygen uptake for a given pulse rate with swimming.

The relationship between maximal oxygen uptake and PWC 170 is shown in Fig. 4. The correlation coefficient value (r) was 0.77. This high correlation of PWC 170 to maximal oxygen uptake in a select group of athletes where the differences between individuals were small is similar to that obtained in a large group of over 500 school children.[4]

Five subjects underwent the extra tests of oxygen uptake to pulse rate relationships with bicycle exercise and swimming. The results of the bicycle test are shown graphically in Figs. 5 and 6. There is an almost linear relationship between oxygen uptake and workload, and between oxygen uptake and pulse rate.

The oxygen uptake/pulse rate relationships during swimming for each of the five subjects are plotted in Fig. 7. A straight line relationship was present between these two variables in four of the five subjects. The mean peak pulse rates were 187 for bicycle exercise and 175 for swimming. The mean peak oxygen uptakes were 56.4 ml./kg. for bicycle work and 49.7 ml./kg. for swimming. Because of technical difficulties of air collection, an absolutely maximal effort was not possible with swimming.

Astrand *et al.*[5] were able to get maximal oxygen uptakes in girls during swimming almost equal to their uptakes with cycling, and we plan to modify our air-collecting apparatus.

DISCUSSION

The mean oxygen uptake/pulse rate ratios, calculated from the above data, are plotted against pulse rate for both the swimming and bicycle exercise in Fig. 8.

It is seen that at lower pulse rates more oxygen is used during swimming. The oxygen/pulse ratio at the slower swimming speeds is greater than that for bicycle exercise.

Our subjects were experienced swimmers, but the breathing apparatus and test procedure were just as new to them as the bicycle exercise, so that the emotional factors should have been similar in the two tests. Why then was swimming associated with a relatively lower pulse rate for a given oxygen uptake?

Factors considered were supine *versus* upright

exercise; a smaller breathing valve with a longer connecting tube; during swimming "weightlessness" produced by water submersion; temperature effects of water; leg *versus* arm plus leg exercise; differences in blood gases; rate and depth of breathing. Another major difference in methodology was that measurements were made after four minutes at each load for cycling, compared to 60 to 120 seconds with each load for swimming. Further investigations are required in this area.

Goff *et al.*[6] and Tuttle and Templin[7] have studied the change in "resting" pulse rate occurring with immersion in water of varying temperatures. In most subjects submerged in water of swimming pool temperature, resting pulse rate declined 10 beats/min. Exercise rates were not obtained. Scholander has studied the heart rate response in diving seals and in man. In the seal, submersion of the nose alone causes a marked and abrupt reflex bradycardia. Cardiac slowing occurs more gradually in man and may be related to changes in blood gases. The relationship of the cardiac slowing under diving conditions to the increased oxygen/pulse ratio of swimming is not clear. Theoretically, cardiac slowing allows more efficient cardiac action with longer diastolic recovery time, which may be an important consideration in reconditioning programs in cardiac patients.

The high pulse rates obtained during competitive water polo reveal that this sport demands from 75 to 100% of maximal effort from the players throughout the game. When it is considered that the oxygen uptake studies during swimming revealed relatively low pulse rates except at near-peak swimming efforts, the rapid heart rates observed during the water polo are indicative of near-maximal metabolic demands.

Sports medicine is looking more and more into physiologic functions in athletes during training and during actual competitive events, and the field of sports medicine is no longer limited to athletic injuries. The elements of suspense and surprise can never be taken away from athletic competition, but the training of athletes is losing its aura of mystery. Development of techniques to measure accurately the physiologic demands of athletic events will help in the development of new methods of athletic training, and in the assessment of conditioning programs.

SUMMARY

A method for monitoring heart rate during water polo has been developed. During the game, rate is seldom below 150 beats/min., often above 170 beats/ min. A comparison of bicycle exercise and swimming showed that there was a difference in the slope of the heart-rate oxygen-uptake curves. There was a slower heart rate for a given oxygen consumption during swimming.

We are indebted to the water-polo players who participated in this work and the Manitoba Water Polo Association for their fullest co-operation. Help with the apparatus was obtained from Mr. Walter Jones of the University of Manitoba and the Maintenance Department, Winnipeg Children's Hospital. We are also indebted to the Physical Education Department, University of Manitoba, for the use of their pool facilities.

REFERENCES

1. WAHLUND, H.: *Acta Med. Scand.,* **132** (Suppl. 215): 1, 1948.
2. CUMMING, G. R. AND CUMMING, P. M.: *Canad. Med. Ass. J.,* 88: 351, 1963.
3. BEHRMANN, V. G. AND HARTMAN, F. W.: *Proc. Soc. Exp. Biol. Med.,* **78:** 412, 1951.
4. CUMMING, G. R.: Unpublished data.
5. ASTRAND, P.-O. *et al.*: *Acta Paediat. (Stockholm),* **52** (Suppl. 147): 1, 1963.
6. GOFF, L. G. *et al.*: *J. Appl. Physiol.,* **9:** 59, 1956.
7. TUTTLE, W. W. AND TEMPLIN, J. L.: *J. Lab. Clin. Med.,* **28:** 271, 1942.

A baseball pitcher's heart rate during actual competition

ALAN STOCKHOLM and HAROLD H. MORRIS

UNTIL RECENT DEVELOPMENTS IN RADIO TELEMETRY the researcher who sought information concerning the physiological responses of the human heart during an activity situation was limited to pre- and post-event recordings (1, 2, 3, 4). This study was conducted to investigate the influences of physical exertion and emotional stress upon the heart rate of a baseball pitcher while actually participating in competition.

The subject was a left-handed Indiania University freshman pitcher, participating in a game against the Indiana State University freshman team. Final score was Indiana University — 8, Indiana State University — 2.

The investigators attached two electrodes on the subject in the manner described by Kozar (2). The transmitter was housed in a belt pocket located at the subject's lower back. Care was taken to provide sufficient play in the electrode lead wires to permit the pitcher complete freedom of motion while throwing. Preparations were completed well before the start of the game to provide time for checking the receiver and recordings, and to allow the subject to participate in normal pregame activities. The subject's fine pitching performance indicates his oblivion to the investigators and the equipment. The Sanborn Telemetry receiver and recorder were sheltered in the dugout

TABLE 1. RUNNING ACCOUNT OF THE EVENTS OF THE BASEBALL

Time	Heart Rate	Event	Time	Heart Rate	Event
12:56	151	Completion of pre-game warm-up	1:28	180	Walking to dugout after hitting D.P. on 1st pitch
12:58	133	Resting in the dugout	1:29	156	Resting in the dugout
1:00	124	Resting in the dugout			
1:01.30	134	Beginning of warm-up			
1:03.10	174	Completion of warm-up	1:31	184	Completion of warm-up, leading 4 to 0
1:04	161	After the 1st pitch			
1:04.10	174	After the 2nd pitch	1:32	184	After the 1st out
1:04.20	180	Prior to the 3rd pitch	1:34	181	After the 2nd out
1:05.25	180	After the 4th pitch, K,* one out	1:35.15	193	After K, 3rd out
1:05.55	174	Prior to 1st pitch, 2nd batter	1:36.15	157	Resting in the dugout
			1:40	134	Beginning of warm-up
1:06.30	180	After pop-up on 2nd pitch, 2 outs	1:42	174	Facing the first batter
1:07.30	181	Prior to 3rd pitch, 3rd batter	1:45	160	After the 2nd out
1:07.50	175	End of inning, walking to the dugout	1:46	137	Resting in the dugout
			1:49	134	Resting in the dugout
			1:52	138	Resting in the dugout
1:08	168	Resting in the dugout	1:53	136	Pitcher on deck
1:09	138	Resting in the dugout	1:53.15	140	Pitcher batting
1:09.30	137	Resting in the dugout	1:53.50	166	Waiting for the 1st pitch
1:12.30	132	Resting in the dugout	1:54	172	After a run to 1st base on a ground-out
1:13	133	Start of warm-up	1:55	170	Resting in the dugout
1:14	168	Prior to the 1st pitch	1:56	174	After the 1st pitch
1:14.20	180	After 1st pitch, flyout	1:58.30	180	After opponents 1st hit, man on 1st, one out
1:15	179	After 2nd pitch, 2nd batter			
1:16	187	After 4th pitch, 2nd batter	1:59	179	Prior to 1st pitch, 3rd batter
1:16.15	182	After 5th pitch, K	1:59.30	180	After pick-off attempt
1:16.45	175	After 1st pitch, foul ball, 3rd batter	2:00.30	162	After 3rd pitch
1:17	170	Prior to 2nd pitch	2:02.20	178	After a double, 1st run for the opponents
1:18	180	Prior to K of 3rd batter			
1:20	157	Resting in the dugout	2:04	168	After 2nd out
1:22	124	Resting in the dugout	2:05	168	After 1st pitch, next batter
1:26	127	Resting in the dugout			
1:27	120	Pitcher on deck	2:06	166	After the 3rd pitch, 5th batter
1:27.20	140	Pitcher batting			
1:27.40	150	Pitcher batting	2:07	170	Prior to the 3rd out

98

Time	Heart Rate	Event	Time	Heart Rate	Event
2:08	150	Resting in the dugout, leading 5 to 1	2:41	170	Completion of warm-up
2:09	127	Resting in the dugout	2:42	174	After the 1st pitch of the inning
2:10.30	132	3rd out, pitcher going to the mound	2:43	179	After a triple, one out
			2:43.30	180	Prior to the 1st pitch, next batter
2:11	136	After the completion of his warm-up	2:44	168	After the 2nd pitch
2:16.20	158	After the 3rd out	2:45	182	Before 1st pitch, 2 outs
			2:45.20	186	After single, 1 run scores
2:17	150	Resting in the dugout	2:46	170	Before 1st pitch, next batter
2:18	126	Resting in the dugout			
2:19	100	Resting in the dugout	2:47	150	Resting in the dugout
2:20	115	Resting in the dugout	2:48	119	Resting in the dugout
2:23	120	Resting in the dugout	2:51	115	Resting in the dugout
			2:56	122	Resting in the dugout
2:23.30	136	Start of the pitcher's warm-up	2:56.40	136	Pitcher on deck
2:25	163	Completion of warm-up	2:57	108	Pitcher on deck
2:25.30	172	After the 2nd pitch, base hit	2:58	133	Pitcher batting
2:26	174	Relief pitcher warming up	2:58.40	173	After the pitcher flied out for the 2nd out
2:27.20	158	After a double play pitch	3:00	164	Resting in the dugout
2:28.30	154	Pause in the action, injured opponent			
2:29	164	After the 3rd pitch, 3rd batter for the 3rd out	3:02	173	After the 2nd pitch
			3:02.20	175	After walking the 1st batter
2:33	148	Pitcher on deck	3:03	173	After the 2nd pitch to the 2nd batter
2:34	139	Pitcher on deck	3:04	168	After the 1st out
2:35	132	Pitcher on 1st after a base hit	3:05	168	After the 2nd out
2:35.30	142	Pitcher standing on 1st	3:05.20	168	After the 3rd out
2:36	160	Pitcher on 1st			
2:37	156	Pitcher on 1st	3:06.20	150	Resting in the dugout Final Score: 8 to 2
2:38	168	Pitcher on 1st	3:07.20	125	Resting in the dugout
2:39	132	Pitcher on 1st	3:08.20	120	Resting in the dugout
			3:09.20	120	Resting in the dugout
2:40	132	3rd out, pitcher warming up			

* K signifies a strike-out

_____ indicates the end of a half inning

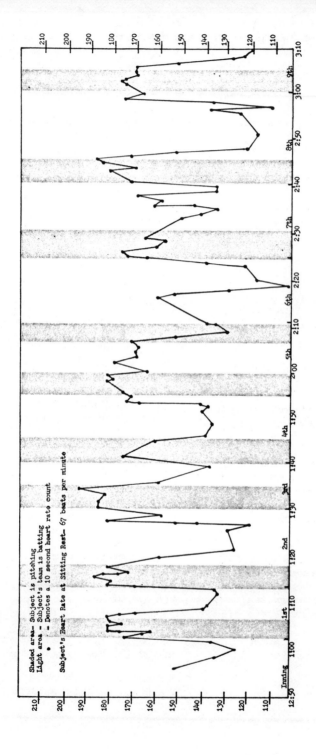

FIGURE 1. *The heart rate, at selected intervals, of a freshman baseball pitcher during a nine-inning game.*

100

approximately 30 yd. from the pitcher's mound and 20 yd. from home plate. Excellent recordings were obtained from as far as second base except during periods of violent movement such as swinging the bat, throwing, and sprinting, when electrical interference from muscular activity disguised the heart rate and accurate readings were unobtainable.

The points plotted in Figure 1 represent 10-sec. counts which were determined by counting R-wave peaks of the ECG. Accuracy was improved by considering the fractional distances before the first and after the last R-wave of a given 10-sec. period.

Discussion

The combination of pre-inning tosses and the excitement of facing the first batter forced the subject's pregame heart rate to 174 beats/min. A peak heart rate of 193 beats/min. was recorded during the third inning of play, and on several occasions before and thereafter the heart rate exceeded 180 beats/min.

Throughout the contest, the subject appeared capable of recovering during the half inning in which his team was at bat, except for the innings in which he was batting or his team was in the process of scoring. Interestingly, even with the longer rests between pitching bouts, the subject's heart rate failed to decline below 100 beats/min.; and on all but three occasions it remained above 120 beats/min. A 5-min. recovery period following the completion of the contest allowed the heart rate to decline to 120.

Baseball may appear to be a relatively nonactive game, but this does not apply to the pitcher. A combination of physical and emotional stress caused the pitcher's heart rate to exceed 180 beats/min. several times during a nine-inning college freshman intercollegiate baseball game. The heart rate failed to decline below 100 for the two hours of competition. The combination of neural and humoral stimuli served to cause the high heart rates.

References

1. Hanson, Dale L. Cardiac response to participation in Little League baseball competition as determined by telemetry. *Research Quarterly* 38:384-88, 1967.
2. Kozar, Andrew J. Telemetered heart rates recorded during gymnastic routines. *Research Quarterly* 34:102-06, 1963.
3. ————, and Hunsicker, Paul. A study of telemetered heart rates during sports participation of young adult men. *Journal of Sports Medicine and Physical Fitness* 3:1-5, 1963.
4. Skubic, Vera, and Hodgkins, Jean. Cardiac response to participation in selected individual and dual sports as determined by telemetry. *Research Quarterly* 36:316-26, 1965.

Techniques for telemetering biopotentials from track athletes during competition

DALE W. SPENCE

WITH THE ADVENT of miniature radiotelemetry instrumentation (5), another dimension of examining the parameters of exercise physiology has been provided. However, the technique of radiotelemetry in monitoring biologic events under dynamic conditions is still very much in the developmental phase. The literature of the past few years has reported a number of investigations of biologic parameters that were monitored during exercise utilizing radiotelemetry instrumentation. This research has been limited to investigations of cardiac response to running events (1, 6, 12, 14, 17), and to specific sports and exercise (2, 3, 4, 8, 9, 15, 16, 18, 19), or to respiration under varying conditions (10). These investigations have been restricted to measurement of one parameter utilizing limited techniques. As investigators continue to seek answers to dynamic biology, standard techniques and new instrumentation need to be developed to enhance the intelligence of biologic monitoring.

The low power transmission range and frequency established by the Federal Communications Commission for biotelemetry instrumentation limits the distance the test subject can be removed from the receiver and display system or recorder. The short range and transmission frequency coupled with the artifacts inherent in the dynamics of exercise seriously tax the system to faithfully reproduce the biologic events. These difficulties are magnified in sports competition where the spectra of biological potential frequencies overlap, where the monitoring of multiple parameters is desirable, and where lightweight instrumentation is at a premium. These conditions, therefore, demand skillful use of the components of the biotelemetry network.

The purpose of this project was to develop a suitable system that could meet the criteria of biologic monitoring of two parameters during dynamic, competitive exercise. It involved the measurement of heart and respiration rates of college athletes during competitive running. Measurements were taken during the running of various sprints and middle-distance races. Competitive track running required that the equipment be lightweight and of a configuration that would not interfere with the performance of the runner. Furthermore, transmission range had to be sufficient so that the signals could be received at a central location from any point along the perimeter of a quarter-mile oval track.

The network consisted of modified instrumentation including a low-power transmitter, a dipole transmitting antenna, a folded dipole receiving antenna, and a biotelemetry receiver. These components were coupled to a display system to record the reproduced physiological data. The miniature transmitter is a lightweight, battery-operated unit designed for short range transmission of biopotentials. It is frequency modulated and operates in the 88-108 megahertz band. It is $32 \times 25 \times 22$ mm in size, weighs 23 g including batteries, and has antenna terminals that permit the use of an accessory dipole antenna to give it an effective range of 400 to 500 ft. The receiver is a line-operated telemetry receiver designed specifically for use with signal-channel biotelemetry transmitters. It has a linear response characteristic essential for the accurate reproduction of original biopotential wave forms and has adjustable filters that allow selective filtering at the output to pass desired information and eliminate unwanted signals or artifacts.[1]

---

[1] E and M Instrument Co., Houston, Texas.

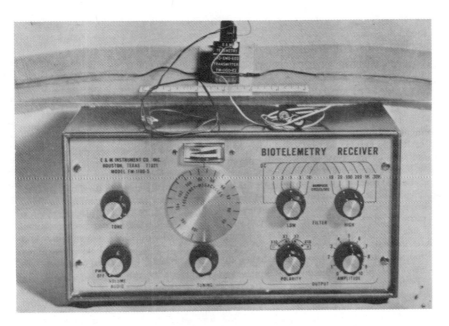

FIGURE 1. *Biotelemetry receiver.*

Because of the small size and weight of the transmitter and because of the low power levels permissable in the 88–108 megahertz band, suitable antennae had to be designed for both the transmitter and receiver to insure adequate reception of signals over the entire circuit of the running track. The transmitter antenna that was used consisted of a one-eighth wave-length dipole mounted on an adhesive-backed foam strip, which in turn was taped to the back of the runner. The receiver antenna consisted of a one-half wave-length folded dipole, vertically polarized, mounted to a 10 ft. mast and located at the center of the running track. A 300-ohm twin-lead transmission cable was used to carry the signal from the antenna to the receiver. From the receiver, the signal output was cabled and then further amplified by a display system.

Transmission of two discrete parameters usually involves either two transmitters or a frequency multiplexing system within a single transmitter. Both of these configurations often sacrifice the lightweight characteristic, which is critical in competitive track running. It was found that a respiration pattern could be modulated with the ECG signal by combining the signals from the electrodes and from a current-biased nasal thermistor. In this configuration, the network utilized a thermistor placed at the nostril to measure resistance change, *viz.*, temperature differentials due to respiration. Both parameters then modulated the same transmitter. The combined signals were separated at the display system by capacitive filtering and separate channeling of the higher frequency ECG wave form signal. The temperature changes were then displayed on a separate channel, which permitted accurate interpretation of respiration rate. In this manner, utilization of the ECG transmitter carrier wave allowed the greatest possible transmission range of respiration.

The "R-wave" of the ECG was used to trigger a cardiotachometer to indicate the consecutive "RR" time intervals directly on the recording. This method of recording gave instantaneous beat-by-beat heart rates that provided rate change information at the exact moment the change occurred, which was displayed both graphically and on the linear scale of the cardiotachometer amplifier.

The transmission band of the transmitter-receiver combination was sufficient to reproduce an ECG of clinical quality. The band-pass filters on the receiver permitted filtering of the very high frequency responses caused by skeletal muscle activity, thus eliminating these undesired potentials that "leak" into the network. However, the high band-pass filters modify the ECG frequency and would not be used for a clinical study of the wave form. The thermistor configuration was highly desirable as it was not susceptible to unwanted movement artifact, which is a bothersome characteristic when using a bellows or impedance pneumograph during exercise.

Electrodes and electrode placement were an important consideration in producing artifact-free wave forms. Since it is not feasible to use standard limb leads during exercise, precordial leads provide a means to monitor rates even though they tend to distort the standard-lead ECG wave form. The electrodes used were nylon silver-silver chloride surface electrodes held in place by double-backed adhesive washers. The surface electrodes were arrangd in an "MX" lead, which is a sternal configuration at the manubrium and xiphoid, to lessen the effect of interference from muscle potentials and chest movement. The "MX" lead provides a sufficient "R-wave" amplitude, which is of primary concern in triggering the cardiotachometer. The electrode lead wires were passed over the shoulder near the neck, then posteriorly to the transmitter, which was taped in place between the scapulae over the thoracic spine. It was essential that the electrode be low mass and securely attached to minimize mechanically produced artifacts due to electrode movement. Best results were obtained when the leads were taped down with some slack near the electrodes, and when the skin was slightly elevated with tape to maintain tautness of subcutaneous tissue, thereby minimizing electrode movement caused by the mass of tissue and electrode. This technique was suggested by Mason and Likar (11) and reduces the D. C. level shift caused by skin and tissue movement reported by Carberry and co-workers (2).

A recent innovation in surface electrode design has some merit because of its extremely low mass. This technique, which was described in a NASA technical brief (13), utilized a spray-on electrode from an air-drying electrically conductive cement mixture that could be applied to the skin to monitor physically active subjects. This very lightweight electrode has no apparent movement independent of the skin, thus eliminating this source of movement artifact. Another type of electrode that has promise for monitoring physically active subjects was reported by Jenkner (7). Although the principal use of this dry Silastic[2] electrode was in electroencephalography, with further experimentation it should be useful during such conditions as were encountered in the present project. The dry electrode provides very low mass and adheres naturally to the skin. It has excellent electrical conducting properties without the use of electrode cream, jelly, or paste. It therefore can be applied quickly and does not irritate the skin or require further maintenance over a prolonged period.

It was found that skin preparation, prior to electrode placement, was extremely important. For example, an area cleaned with acetone and alcohol only had a skin-electrode impedance of 80 kilohms, which prevented effective use of the frequency multiplex thermistor-bias technique. When the skin was lightly abraded in preparation for electrode application, the skin-electrode impedance dropped to 1 kilohm, which resulted in an ECG-pneumotach recording with little artifact.

[2] Dow Corning Center for Aid to Medical Research, Midland, Michigan.

References

1. BOWLES, CHARLES J., and SIGERSETH, PETER O. Telemetered heart rate responses to pace patterns in the one mile run. *Research Quarterly* 39:36-46, 1968.
2. CARBERRY, WILLIAM J.; TOLLES, WALTER E.; and FREIMAN, ALVIN H. A system for monitoring the ECG under dynamic conditions. *Aerospace Medicine* 31: 131-37, 1960.

3. HANSON, DALE L. Cardiac response to participation in Little League baseball competition as determined by telemetry. *Research Quarterly* 38: 384-88, 1967.
4. HANSON, J. S., and TABAKIN, B. S. Electrocardiographic telemetry in skiers. *New England Journal of Medicine* 271: 181-85, 1964.
5. HOLTER, N. J. Radioelectrocardiography: A new technique for cardiovascular studies. *Annals of the New York Academy of Science* 65: 913-23, 1957.
6. HOWARD, GORDON E.; BLYTH, CARL S.; and THORNTON, WILLIAM E. Effects of warm-up on the heart rate during exercise. *Research Quarterly* 37: 360-67, 1966.
7. JENKNER, F. L. A new electrode material for multipurpose bio-medical application. *Electroencephalography and Clinical Neurophysiology* 23: 570-71, 1967.
8. KOZAR, ANDREW J. Telemetered heart rates recorded during gymnastic routines. *Research Quarterly* 34: 102-106, 1963.
9. ————, and HUNSICKER, PAUL. A study of telemetered heart rates during sports participation of young adult men. *Journal of Sports Medicine and Physical Fitness* 3: 1-5, 1963.
10. KROBATH, H., and REID, C. A new method for the continuous recording of the volume of inspiration and expiration under widely varying conditions. *American Journal of Medical Electronics* 3: 105-09, 1964.
11. MASON, ROBERT E., and LIKAR, IVAN. A new system of multiple-lead exercise electrocardiography. *American Heart Journal* 71: 196-205, 1966.
12. McARDLE, WILLIAM D.; GOGLIA, GUIDO F.; and PATTI, ANTHONY V. Cardiac response to running events. *Journal of Applied Physiology* 23: 566-70, 1967.
13. NATIONAL AERONAUTICS AND SPACE ADMINISTRATION. NASA Tech. Brief #66-10649. Washington, D. C.: NASA, December 1960.
14. ORBAN, W. A. R., AND OTHERS. Heart rate responses to interval running using radiotelemetry. *Journal of Sports Medicine and Physical Fitness* 3: 252-53, 1963.
15. ROSE, KENNETH D., and DUNN, LOWELL F. A study of heart function in athletes by telemetered electrocardiography. *Proceedings of the 5th Annual Conference on the Medical Aspects of Sports.* AMA, 1963.
16. ROSENBLAT, V. V. Heart rate in man during natural muscular activity (data obtained by dynamic radiotelemetry). *Federation Proceedings.* (Trans. Suppl.) 22:T761-66, 1963.
17. SKUBIC, VERA, and HILGENDORF, JANE. Anticipatory, exercise, and recovery heart rates of girls as affected by four running events. *Journal of Applied Physiology* 19: 853-56, 1964.
18. SKUBIC, VERA, and HODGKINS, JEAN. Cardiac response to participation in selected individual and dual sports as determined by telemetry. *Research Quarterly* 36: 316-26, 1965.
19. ————. Relative strenuousness of selected sports as performed by women. *Research Quarterly* 38:305-13, 1967.

The EEG in the Traumatic Encephalopathy of Boxers

J. JOHNSON

The traumatic encephalopathy of boxers which gives rise to 'punch drunkenness' [MARTLAND, 1928], is due to the cumulative effects of repetitive brain trauma received during a boxer's career [MAWDSLEY and FERGUSON, 1963]. In some cases permanent brain damage results [BOWMAN and BLAU, 1960] whilst in others a progressive degenerative process is induced which continues even after an active boxing career has been abandoned [CRITCHLEY, 1957; SPILLANE, 1962]. It was not surprising, therefore, that clinicians turned to the investigation of the electrical activity of the brain in order to try and detect the encephalopathy in its early sub-clinical forms.

BUSSE and SILVERMAN [1952] first carried out routine electroencephalograms on boxers in the state of Colorado after they had had a knock out in the ring and compared them with a control group of normals. Although they demonstrated a high incidence of abnormality (37 %), they were unable to correlate the degree of electrical abnormality with features of the boxers' fighting history. They commented that many of the boxers had 'aggressive personalities' and that the EEG abnormalities may be related to this personality abnormality rather than to intrinsic brain damage. LARSSON [1954], used the EEG to study the effects upon cerebral function of individual bouts. He took records 15 to 30 minutes after a fight in amateur boxers and found generalized flattening of the record with irregular slow activity in 13 %: the figure rose to 30 % if the boxer had sustained a 'knock out' blow during the bout. KAPLAN and BOWDER [1954] reported the EEG findings of over 1,000 professional boxers together with ringside observations on the intensity of the fight. The authors, a neurologist and a New York State Boxing Commissioner paid only 'lip service' to the punch drunk syndrome and could find no significant change in the EEG after a bout. They did admit, however, that poorly rated fighters, ('sluggers'), had more disorganized records than did competent boxers. PAMPUS and GROTE [1956], carried out EEGs on 250 active and 17 retired boxers. They found a correlation between the frequency of abnormal EEGs and the number of fights; after three or more fights in one week the resting EEG was abnormal in 42 %. They noted slow resolution of these abnormalities, particularly in juveniles, and felt that the boxers should be excluded from boxing until the EEG returned to normal.

CRITCHLEY [1957] stated that minor, non-specific, EEG changes were commonly seen in boxers whilst more disorganized records were found in those suffering from a 'punch drunk' state. He expressed the hope that the EEG might be used to detect and screen boxers from the early phases of the encephalopathy. Since then no detailed studies of the EEG in this disorder have been reported.

The psychiatric aspects of the encephalopathy of boxers were recently described in 17 ex-boxers who were referred to a hospital because they were thought to be suffering from this disorder [JOHNSON, 1968]: the EEG, neuroradiological and psychometric findings were also reported. The EEG findings are here described in detail and an attempt is made to evaluate their diagnostic value in relation to the other forms of investigation, by correlating the degree of abnormality to the severity of the clinical syndrome.

Results

EEG findings

Bipolar, scalp EEGs were carried out in the 17 cases of the series; abnormal records were present in 10. These were severely abnormal in one case, moderately abnormal in four cases and borderline abnormal in five. Two main types of abnormal record were recognised:

1. a flat, low voltage record with minimal (below 25 μV) or absent alpha rhythm throughout the record (fig. 1), was present in three records (1, 3, 7);

2. an alpha dominant record with randomly occurring mixtures of slow and intermediate slow background activity was present in 7 records (fig. 2), (2, 6, 9, 14, 15, 16, 17).

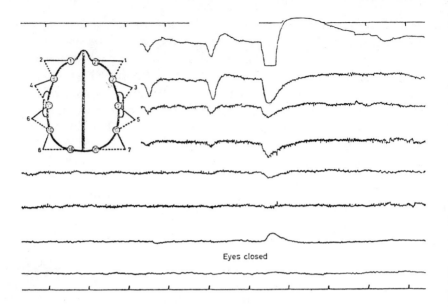

Fig. 1. J. B. 6-3-63. Flat, low voltage record with minimal (below 25 μV) or absent alpha rhythm.

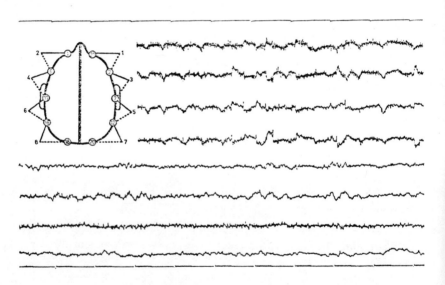

Fig. 2. Th. M. 25-5-65. Alpha dominant record with randomly occurring mixtures of slow and intermediate slow background activity.

All the records were examined 'blind' without knowledge of the clinical details of the cases and were assessed numerically along four different parameters, viz., abnormalities in the dominant rhythm, the background rhythms, transient abnormal rhythms and abnormalities produced by activation procedures (hyperventilation and photicstimulation). Each parameter was assessed as

0 = no abnormality
1 = mild abnormality
2 = moderate abnormality
3 = severe abnormality

The maximal total score for abnormal record was 12: summated scores are shown in table I.

Table I. Rating scores of severity of clinical state and investigations

Case No.	Neuro-logical	Psychiatric	Total clinical rating	AEG (0–3)	Psycho-metric tests (0–3)	EEG rating (0–12)
1	4	4	8	3	3	3
2	3	1	4	0	0	2
3	0.5	1	1.5	2	1	3
4	0	0	0	0	0	0
5	0	1	1	–	–	0
6	4	3	7	2	2	2
7	1	0	1	2	2	2
8	2.5	3	5.5	2	0	0
9	2	4	6	2	2	2
10	1.5	3	4.5	2	2	0
11	1	1	2	2	–	0
12	3	1	4	2	0	0
13	2	1	3	2	1	0
14	0.5	0	0.5	2	1	7
15	3	2	5	2	3	2
16	3	3	6	–	3	3
17	1	3	4	1	2	4

Neuroradiological findings
Lumbar air encephalography (AEG) was carried out in 15 of the 17 cases and evidence of brain damage demonstrated in 13. ISHERWOOD *et al.* [1966] described the main neuroradiological abnormalities in this traumatic encephalopathy, the specific features of which had first been described by SPILLANE [1962]. Three abnormal radiological findings were assessed as present or absent from the neuroradiologist's reports viz. communicating cavum septii pellucidii, cortical or cerebellar atrophy and ventricular dilatation. A maximal rating of 3 was therefore possible if all abnormalities were present in the AEG (table I).

Psychometric findings
Psychometric tests of brain damage (Wechsler Adult Intelligence Scale, Benton Visual Retention Test and an auditory Word Learning Test), were carried out in 15 cases by a clinical psychologist and were abnormal in 11. As these tests measure different aspects of brain damage a single point was allocated for evidence of abnormality in any one test (table I).

Clinical findings
The clinical manifestations of the traumatic encephalopathy vary widely in severity. In some cases they are mild and non-progressive (Cases 5, 7, 14) whilst in others they are severe and progressive (1, 8, 9, 16). Neurological features were numerically rated according to the presence of pyramidal, extrapyramidal, cerebellar signs, epilepsy and impotence. Psychiatric features were enumerated according to the presence or absence of an amnestic state, dementia, morbid jealousy syndrome, psychosis, explosive personality reactions. A total clinical score was obtained by summating the psychiatric and neurological abnormalities to give a maximum of 10 possible symptoms (table I).

The investigations and the clinical state were then arranged in rank order according to the degree of severity. Each investigation was then correlated in turn with the severity of the clinical state and Spearman's rank correlation coefficient calculated (table II).

Discussion

An EEG abnormality of a non-specific nature was present in 60 % of the patients in this series. The low voltage 'flat' record, present in three cases

Table II. Correlations between clinical state and investigations

	Clinical state		
	AEG	Psychometric	EEG
No. Subjects	15	15	17
Spearman's Rank Correlation Coefficient	0.6187	0.5777	0.1103
't' test (N-2)	2.83	2.5	0.42
Percentage	1–2 %	2–5 %	>10 %

(1, 3, 7) has been previously described in patients suffering from Huntington's chorea and dementia [MARGERISON and SCOTT, 1965]. GORDON and SIM [1967] have also noted a high incidence of this type of record in patients with presenile dementia of the Alzheimer type. The EEG abnormality in the remaining seven cases affected the background rhythms and occurred randomly except in one case (14) where there was a localized focal abnormality in one parietal area.

Although the overall incidence of EEG abnormalities in the traumatic encephalopathy is high, the correlation between the severity of the clinical syndrome and the degree of disorganization of the EEG is poor ($r = 0.1103$). On the other hand evidence of brain damage on the air encephalogram shows a high correlation with the degree of severity of the clinical syndrome ($r = 0.6187$) whilst evidence of brain damage on psychometric tests showed a significant although lower order of correlation ($r = 0.5777$). The lesions responsible for the encephalopathy are probably located in two main areas [JOHNSON, 1968]. Those responsible for the neurological features are in the upper brain stem whilst those related to the psychiatric features are in the hippocampal-fornical system. As the scalp EEG predominantly reflects neural disorganization in the cerebral cortex it is not surprising that there is a low level of correlation between the EEG abnormalities and the severity of the clinical syndrome since the responsible lesions are largely subcortical.

Three cases (1, 16, 17) showed definite evidence of progressive, intellectual deterioration i. e. dementia, whilst a fourth case (15) was showing evidence of early dementia at follow-up; all had abnormal EEGs. Although the EEG is frequently abnormal in patients suffering from dementia, most investigators have found the level of correlation to be low between the degree of dementia and the severity of the EEG abnormality. TURTON and WARREN [1960] in their study of dementia over the age of 60, concluded that the EEG was of little value in distinguishing dementia from functional psychosis. GORDON and SIM [1967] similarly found a poor correlation between the EEG and the 'intellectual component' of a differential assessment of dementia in the presenium.

Transient abnormalities in the EEG immediately after a boxing bout [LARSSON et al., 1954] reveal temporary neuronal disorganization particularly when the boxer has been involved in a 'knock down'. The EEG might be used as a convenient method of deciding when such disorganization has resolved and when a fighter can safely resume his boxing activities. The use of the routine EEG as a screening procedure for the detection of the incipient traumatic encephalopathy therefore appears to be limited in view of the low level of correlation between the severity of the syndrome and the EEG abnormality. Psychometric testing and air encephalopathy (where justified) offer more accurate evidence of the severity of the traumatic encephalopathy.

The findings of this investigation must, however, be interpreted with reservation. Visual analysis of EEG records by clinicians combined with simple computations of their abnormalities are of limited value. Whilst the changes in a single record as in this series may be normal or only minimally abnormal, the changes observed in serial records may be more significant. The application of wave analysis and computation to serial records on boxers may well reveal early and more significant evidence of an insidious encephalopathy than isolated records can do. Although the EEG is revealed in this investigation as poorly correlated with the severity of the traumatic encephalopathy of boxers, this is probably due to the limitations imposed by present clinical methods of interpretation.

Acknowledgments

I wish to thank Dr. IAN ISHERWOOD for his help in the neuroradiological aspects of this investigation and Mr. J. C. KENNA for the psychological testing.

Summary

The EEG findings in 17 ex-boxers with evidence of traumatic encephalopathy are reported. Two main abnormalities were seen viz. flat, low voltage records in 3 cases; diffuse slow and intermediate slow background rhythms in alpha dominant records in 7 cases. Correlations between the degree of EEG abnormality, psychometric tests and neuroradiological findings showed the EEG to have the lowest correlation. This is probably due to the limits imposed by visual analysis on isolated records. Serial EEG records during the active careers of boxers would probably be of more value in detecting the insidious encephalopathy.

References

BOWMAN, K. M. and BLAU, A.: Psychotic states following head injury; in S. BROCK, Injuries of tle brain and spinal cord (Cassell, London 1960).

BUSSE, E. W. and SILVERMAN, A. J.: EEG changes in professional boxers. J. Amer. med. Ass. *149:* 1522 (1952).

CRITCHLEY, M.: Medical aspects of boxing. Brit. med. J. *i:* 357 (1957).

GORDON, E. B. and SIM, M.: EEG in presenile dementia. J. Neurol. Neurosurg. Psychiat. *30:* 285 (1967).

ISHERWOOD, I.; MAWDSLEY, C. and FERGUSON, F. R.: Pneumoencephalographic changes in boxers. Acta radiol., Stockh. *5:* 654 (1966).

JOHNSON, J.: Organic psychosyndromes due to boxing. Brit. J. Psychiat. *115:* 45 (1969).

KAPLAN, H. A. and BOWDER, J.: Observations on the clinical and brain wave patterns of professional boxers. J. Amer. med. Ass. *156:* 1138 (1954).

LARSSON, L. E. and MELIN, K. A.: Acute head injuries in boxers. Acta psychiat. neurol. scand., Suppl. 95 (1954).

MARGERISON, J. H. and SCOTT, D. F.: Huntington's chorea: EEG and neuropathological findings. Electroenceph. clin. Neurophysiol. *19:* 314 (1965).

MARTLAND, H. S.: Punch drunk. J. Amer. med. Ass. *91:* 1103 (1928).

MAWDSLEY, C. and FERGUSON, F. R.: Neurological disease in boxers. Lancet *ii:* 795 (1963).

PAMPUS, F. and GROTE, W.: Electroencephalographic and clinical findings in boxers. Arch. Psychiat. Nevenkr. *194:* 152 (1956).

SPILLANE, J. D.: Five boxers. Brit. med. J. *ii:* 1205 (1962).

TURTON, E. C. and WARREN, P. K. G.: Dementia: a clinical and EEG study of 274 patients over the age of 60. J. ment. Sci. *106:* 1493 (1960).

Diving and Medicine

BLAKE W. MEADOR, M.D.

THOUSANDS OF PEOPLE have taken up skin diving which requires only simple mask, fins, and snorkle. This type of diving is self-limited. However, the scuba divers (using Self-Contained Underwater Breathing Apparatus) are the true divers.

The early growth of scuba diving was particularly slow, because the sport was a "war baby". It was born in 1943 when Jacques Yves Cousteau of the French Navy, and an engineer named Emile Gagnon used secondhand ideas to perfect a breathing regulator that enabled ordinary men to go below with a tankful of adventure on their backs. Since 1950 more than 600,000 regulators have been sold in the United States, most of them to folks who a few years ago never dreamed of going into this unreal world.

Panel Symposium on Environmental Cardio-Pulmonary Physiology in Sports Diving, Weightlessness, and Altitude Flying—A.M.A. (Chest Division) Chicago 1966.

It is only with the coming of the Explorers Club that the sport has really zoomed. On Grand Bahama the novice who makes satisfactory progress can, in the matter of a week, enjoy the shallow reefs and also wander in safe company into the spectacular twilight farther down. The Club will supply guides for fully experienced divers to the 150 foot level, a short way into the Narcosis Zone.

Today this sport (skin and scuba diving) in the United States is assumed to have over seven million members and of these four million use scuba equipment. However, the fourth leading type of fatal accident in this country is drowning—approximately 7,000 deaths are reported a year. This emphasizes the point that the very best equipment that can be obtained should be used. Beware of using homemade equipment or any type of rebreathing apparatus. The rebreathing apparatus is only used with pure oxygen by the military services especially during war time. This type of equipment is used by the military to prevent the "tell-tale" bubbles from reaching the surface of the water.

Pure oxygen when used with the rebreathing equipment is more risky and toxic than compressed air. Ten minutes at 40 feet depth is the maximum safe time allowable with oxygen. In sport diving compressed air is used, because it is much safer, less expensive, and the allowable time under water is much longer. Air is 78% nitrogen, 21% oxygen, carbon dioxide .035, and other inert gases .97%. To avoid carbon dioxide and carbon monoxide poisoning be sure to fill the tanks with an electrical operated compressor. Never use a gasoline operated compressor and never use a compressor lubricated with oil.

By skin diving, the Korean and Japanese women have made a living from what they recovered from the ocean floor for centuries. Through life-long practice it is amazing what they can accomplish. The lung volumes and alveolar gases during actual dives were studied in the Korean diving women. The average velocities of descent and ascent was 0.6 foot per second. The maximum depth and duration of dive observed was 17 feet and 82 seconds respectively. However, typical sustained diving activity is to a depth of five feet for 30 seconds; averaging 60 dives per hour. The Japanese as a rule, work in pairs, the man handling the boat and the woman diving. This diving pattern, or assisted dives of the Japanese last 60 seconds and reach a depth of about 20 feet. Prior to diving the lung is filled to 85% of vital capacity; about 700 CC of this gas is lost upon return to the surface. Hyperventilation before diving reduces the PCO_2 to 28. As you would expect at the bottom, the fractional composition of oxygen as well as carbon dioxide is less than before the dive, indicating that both gases are removed by the circulation. Bottom O_2 pressure is high due to compression, but falls rapidly upon ascent. The compression of the gases accounts for the reversal of CO_2 transport; upon return to the surface CO_2 leaves the blood and reaches normal values.

In sport diving fifty feet should be your maximum depth; at a lower level you would find very little sunlight. Most experts agree that a descent of from 15-30 feet, just beyond the shore line, can bring you into contact with this new and ever changing world. In skin diving the recommended beginner diving limit is 25 feet; intermediate and spear fish diving limit 50 feet; one hundred feet is considered the maximum for expert skin divers; beginners in scuba diving should be limited to 35-40 feet, and for expert scuba divers 125 feet. For water temperature above 75 degrees-F., no special suit is required; for temperatures 60-75 degrees-F., woolen underwear; 30-60 degrees-F., wet or dry suit and for temperatures below 30 degrees F., combination of wet and dry suits.

Don't let underwater distances fool you; for example, a three foot fish at a distance of 12 feet, would appear to be four feet long and nine feet in actual distance. Remember sound travels underwater at 4900 feet per second, also one 72 cubic foot tankful of air will supply the scuba diver for 30 minutes at a depth of 66 feet. The writer insists on the "Buddy System"—never sports dive alone—your "swimming buddy" would be life saving if and when you get in trouble.

Roughly we might say that for every one foot depth of water there is approximately one-half pound increase in pressure or thoracic squeeze. At sea level our vital capacity would be five liter—the pressure 14.7 —one atmosphere (Psi)—one tank of compressed air would last 90 minutes—at 33 feet, 29.4, 2 atm. (Psi)—you would have the equivalent of one-half tank compressed air, good for 45 minutes. At 66 feet, 44.1 pounds, 3 atm. (Psi), one-third tank compressed air, good for 30 minutes—at 99 feet, 58.8 pounds, 4 atm. (Psi), one-quarter tank compressed air good for 23 minutes— at 132 feet, 73.8 pounds, 5 atm. (Psi), one-fifth tank compressed air good for 18 minutes. It would be wise to write the Navy Medicine Department, c/o Submarine and Diving School, to obtain the charts which states the maximum length of time that may be spent under water. If that time limit is exceeded for a stated depth then the diver must be put in a compression chamber. There is no reason for such a problem developing, but as we all know, some people think the rules are made for other people. Each sports diving club should write the Navy Medical Department and determine where the nearest portable compression chamber is or would be available. Remember that nitrogen is cumulative, therefore the charts showing the maximum time allowable underwater (stated depth), would be for a 12-hour period. If you desire, recall Boyles Law and its practical application in scuba diving (the volume of a gas varies inversely as the pressure, if temperature is constant).

Many problems develop in ascent; the diver must not ascend faster than 50-60 feet per minute; do not get panicky and hold your breath. You must exhale freely as you ascend; this will prevent "bubbles" or nitrogen retention. Always take a seasick tablet before diving. Seasickness is more prevalent than realized, and vomiting would be fatal.

A physical examination should be a must before taking up skin or scuba diving. The diver must be able to withstand heavy exertion; have no psychiatric condition, the chest must be x-rayed, not overweight, no ear disease or perforation of the drum, no evidence of sinus disease, vision and hearing must be normal and no cardio-vascular problems. To take up sports diving for the excitement or thrill should be unthought of and very foolish. And never forget, when you go diving, have a pal or buddy with you.

Skin diving and scuba diving is one of the last uncrowded sports open to you. You move through the water in a state of weightlessness that is exhilarating to both mind and body. There is a world down there that staggers the imagination. A vast silent world that is timeless in its beauty. Possibly you may wish to discover the answer to the question "What's down there?"

REFERENCES

U.S. Bureau of Medicine and Surgery, Navy Department.

U.S. Bureau of Ships, Navy Department. Bureau of Ships, Diving Manual.

U.S. Bureau of Naval Personnel, Navy Dept., Submarine Medicine Practice.

George Smith, M.D., Aberdeen, Scotland, 1963.

Handbook of Physiology, Section 3. Respiration Volume II, Editors Wallace C. Fenn & Hermann Rahn.

Diving Medicine. E. H. Lamphier. New England J. M., 1957.

RUNNING TOWARDS OLYMPUS

EDWARD BYRNE-QUINN
ROBERT F. GROVER.

SIR,—In the last paragraph of your leader (Oct. 12, p. 816) you say: " Systemic hypoxia has a constrictive effect on the small vessels on the arterial side of the pulmonary circulation, because of the hypoxic mixed venous blood, rather than the hypoxic alveolar air.'· In the symposium [1] which you give as a reference, we are unable to find any corroboration of this statement. Rather we find several workers who state clearly that hypoxic alveolar air is in fact the important stimulus—e.g., J. M. Bishop on p. 137, L. Reid on p. 157 citing von Euler and Liljestrand,[2] and D. Heath on pp. 168–169 again citing von Euler and Liljestrand.[2] Furthermore, there is considerable evidence that lowering the mixed-venous oxygen tension, while alveolar oxygen tension remains high, does *not* produce pulmonary hypertension.[3][4] Severe anæmia is not associated with pulmonary hypertension,[5][6] yet the mixed-venous oxygen tension is abnormally low at all times.

Regarding exercise, you state: " There seems to be no information about whether or not pulmonary hypertension occurs in exercise at sea level, but it seems inescapable that moving to 7450 feet will increase the possibility of this happening." In normal subjects the mean pulmonary-artery pressure has been shown to be normal during exercise [7] or very slightly increased (by 5 mm. Hg) compared with rest, but remaining constant at different work-loads.[8] Pulmonary vascular resistance, on average, decreased in these studies, especially at high work-loads. In *athletes*, at maximal exercise (1600 k.p.m. per minute), the mean pulmonary-artery pressure has been shown to be higher than in normals in proportion to a higher pulmonary wedge pressure. The decrease in pulmonary resistance followed the same regression line as found for normal subjects.[9] Therefore pulmonary vasoconstriction does not seem to occur in normal subjects or athletes during exercise when the mixed-venous oxygen tension is low.

In a study from this laboratory,[10] eight normal subjects had full hæmodynamic measurements performed at rest and during 600 k.p.m. per minute exercise both at sea-level and after ten days at 3100 m. altitude (10,200 feet). Both pulmonary-artery pressure and pulmonary vascular resistance remained within normal limits. In our opinion it is doubtful that there has been any problem of pulmonary hypertension at the lower altitude of 2270 m. (7450 feet) at Mexico City.

1. Form and Function in the Human Lung (edited by G. Cumming and L. B. Hunt). Edinburgh, 1968.
2. von Euler, V. S., Liljestrand, G. *Acta physiol. scand.* 1946, **12**, 301.
3. Reeves, J. T., Leathers, J. E., Eiseman, B., Spencer, F. C. *Medna thorac.* 1962, **19**, 561.
4. Vogel, J. H. K., in Normal and Abnormal Pulmonary Circulation (edited by R. F. Grover); p. 387. New York, 1963.
5. Leight, L., Snider, T. H., Clifford, G. O., Hellems, H. K. *Circulation*, 1954, **10**, 653.
6. Roy, S. B., Bhatia, M. L., Mathur. V. S., Virmani, S. *ibid.* 1963, **28**, 346.
7. Bevegård, S., Holmgren, A., Jonsson, B. *Acta physiol. scand.* 1960, **49**, 279.
8. Holmgren, A., Jonsson, B., Sjöstrand, T. *ibid.* p. 343.
9. Bevegård, S., Holmgren, A., Jonsson, B. *ibid.* 1963, **57**, 26.
10. Alexander, J. K., Hartley, L. H., Modelski, M., Grover, R. F. *J. Appl. Physiol.* 1967, **23**, 849.

Cardiovascular adaptations in diving mammals

Harald T. Andersen, Ph.D.

The seals (Pinnipedia) and the whales (Cetacea) are highly developed animals. The level of organization of their central nervous systems, especially that of the cetaceans, is unsurpassed among animals. The metabolic processes of their organisms proceed at a high rate, thus, seals and whales maintain body temperatures of 35 to 38° C.

Such specialized organisms are usually highly vulnerable to asphyxia. Acute respiratory arrest in man and most other air-breathing vertebrates causes great discomfort, loss of consciousness, and convulsive efforts to breathe. If breathing remains obstructed, death is certain within a few minutes. However, the diving vertebrates are able to remain submerged for prolonged periods of time (15 minutes to 2 hours) without showing any motor disability upon emersion, and yet, they are equipped with essentially the same respiratory and circulatory organs as their terrestrial relatives.[1] Moreover, it has been recorded that the Weddel seal, *Leptonychotes weddelli*, may dive as deep as 600 M,[2] and indirect evidence indicates that the sperm whale, *Physeter catadon*, may descend to approximately 1,000 M.[3] These depths are the deepest on record, but there are numerous reports in the literature of various species of vertebrate divers descending several hundred meters down in the oceans.[4] The ability of homeothermic vertebrate divers to descend to great depths and remain under water for extended periods of time present the comparative physiologist with two formidable questions. These problems have been thoroughly investigated over the past 30 years, and the results are such that they may be of general interest to physiologists and physicians alike.

Prolonged diving

Since seals and whales are unable to extract oxygen from the water by means of accessory respiratory organs, they must depend on the oxygen stores within the body for aerobic metabolism when they are submerged. Estimates of the total amount of stored oxygen in diving mammals have shown that the oxygen deposits are larger in divers than in nondivers, but nevertheless are insufficient to maintain an aerobic metabolism at the prediving rate during a long submersion. The possibility of a switching from aerobic to anaerobic metabolism during diving has been suggested by several authors,[5,6] and investigated with various methods. Continuous registrations of oxygen consumption before and after diving have shown that the excess intake of oxygen after a prolonged, quiet, and restrained dive is much less than would have

121

been expected.[7] Direct temperature measurements have also shown that the total energy metabolism is lowered in diving seals.[8] For these reasons it seems safe to conclude that an increase in anaerobic processes does not compensate for the lack of oxygen.

Even 30 years ago, Irving[9] realized that the vertebrate divers do not carry enough oxygen to perform prolonged submergence. He pointed out that the brain and the heart are easily and irreparably damaged by lack of oxygen, asserted that the muscles may be left hypoxic for relatively long periods of time without ill effects, and concluded that, when no chemical or physical processes seem to adapt the vertebrate divers for submergence, one should consider whether reflex adjustments do. Irving suggested that the available oxygen is reserved for the brain and the heart by a differential distribution of the circulating blood. Later research has verified practically every one of his predictions.

The French physiologist Bert[10] reported a reflex adjustment to diving almost 100 years ago. He discovered that the heart rate of ducks fell upon submergence from more than 100 beats per minute to less than fifteen. Bert's observation has been confirmed in every diving vertebrate investigated. This phenomenon takes place in nondivers and in man as well, but it is not as strikingly developed in terrestrial animals as in aquatic ones.

The diving bradycardia is due to vagal inhibition, as was first shown in ducks by Richet.[11] His finding has been confirmed by several authors who work with different vertebrate divers.[12-16] Diving bradycardia is due to prolongation of the diastole; the electrocardiogram (ECG) is thus characterized by a very marked increase of the T-Q interval. Other prominent changes in the ECG include progressive lengthening of the P-R interval with eventual disappearance of the P wave. The T wave is usually elevated and peaked; sometimes it appears diphasic or inverted.

The ECG changes also suggest hyperkalemia, and it has been shown that the concentration of potassium in plasma may increase as much as threefold in ducks during submersions which last for 8 minutes. The nervous influence, however, seems by far the more important, for the P wave reappears in emersion in spite of maximally elevated plasma potassium, and the P-R interval is then shortened in correspondence with a postdiving tachycardia. The T wave, on the other hand, remains elevated and peaked for several minutes.[17]

The bradycardia, although extreme, does not explain how diving animals are able to endure long periods of underwater exposures. In fact, its significance was not appreciated until almost 75 years after its discovery when Irving, Scholander, and Grinnell[18] studied the regulation of arterial blood pressure in diving seal. They found that the pressure in the femoral artery remained near the normal level in spite of an extreme bradycardia, whereas the pressure in a small artery in one of the flippers fell abruptly upon submersion. Likewise, marked vasoconstriction took place in mesenterial vessels. Widespread vasoconstriction was evidenced also by the observations that: (1) the myoglobin was completely reduced at a time when the arterial blood was still 50 per cent saturated; (2) the amount of lactic acid in the blood increased very little or not at all during diving, but rose markedly upon emersion; (3) a wound in skin or in muscles would bleed profusely before and after submersion, whereas during diving no bleeding occurred.

These 3 findings were interpreted to mean that the muscles are effectively shunted out of the circulation when the animal is submerged.

Data obtained in the duck show that cutaneous and intestinal circulations are suspended in diving birds,[19] and measurements in seals[20] and ducks[21] have revealed that the urine formation stops upon water immersion, which indicates a greatly reduced renal blood flow. Recently, Elsner and associates[22] have reported a stoppage of flow of blood in the abdominal aorta and renal artery of submerged harbor seals. The blood flow in the common carotid artery was reduced, but sustained at a higher level than in the other arteries mentioned. It thus seems that all vascular beds except the brain and the heart are constricted during diving. In this way the diving vertebrates reserve their limited oxygen stores for the tissues most easily damaged by lack of oxygen, whereas the rest of the organism is left with little or no oxygen at all during submersion.

The results obtained on diving vertebrates have stirred the interest in cardiovascular adjustments in general and a number of recent studies have verified that these responses to underwater conditions take place in terrestrial animals and in man under normal and pathologic conditions as well. The same types of cardiovascular reflexes that are so conspicuously exhibited by diving vertebrates have been encountered in the human fetus at birth, in patients with myocardial infarction, ventricular aneurisms, coronary arteriosclerosis, after hemorrhage, and in patients with severe pulmonary insufficiency. Pertinent references to the literature on this subject have been included in several recent reviews.[1,22-25]

Deep diving

During the last decade, skin and scuba diving have become very popular. With the number of amateur divers increasing, the accident rate has increased greatly, and the symptoms and causes of injury from deep dives have become generally known. Considering our knowledge of diving times and depths in the aquatic mammals one may wonder why these animals apparently never incur at least two types of injury common among human divers, namely, lung squeeze and caisson disease (bends; decompression illness).

When a diver descends, the pressure increases with approximately one atmosphere for every 10 meters. The tissues and the body fluids are practically incompressible, but the gas phase within the body will undergo volume reduction. Also, the increasing ambient pressure will cause additional amounts of the lung gases to be dissolved in the blood.

It is probably fair to assume that any intestinal gas is compressed according to the increase in hydrostatic pressure, since the soft abdominal wall will readily transmit the ambient pressure to the deeper parts of the body. The thorax, on the other hand, may resist increasing pressure to some extent. In this case, the diaphragm would bulge into the thorax and blood would distend the heart and the blood vessels in response to the pressure difference between the thorax cavity and the surroundings.[7] But if the thorax is fairly rigid, as it is for instance in humans, the gas pressure in the lungs and airways will eventually fall below the ambient pressure. At this point, lung squeeze with pulmonary edema and rupture of the capillaries may develop in human skin divers. Such a condition has not been observed in marine mammals. This may be explained by the marked flexibility of the thorax of marine mammals. Whereas the thorax of most terrestrial mammals is rather rigid, and the tidal volume is usually only a fraction of the total lung volume, the lungs of marine mammals may become practically atelectatic without losing contact with the chest wall.[7] This flexibility of the thorax allows certain marine mammals to empty the lungs down to the dead space in expiration; in fact, it has been shown that the tidal volume very nearly equals the lung volume in the bottlenose (*Tursiops truncatus*).[26] Thus, one may postulate that the lung air in whales is compressed during submersion in accordance with the hydrostatic pressure.[7] Therefore, pressure differences may not develop in diving whales, and lung squeezes are consequently never incurred.

The flexible properties of the thorax of seals and whales and the corresponding collapse of their lungs during deep dives are important also when the possibility of caisson disease in aquatic mammals is considered. When the animal leaves the surface and descends to great depths, the ambient hydrostatic pressure is readily transmitted to all parts of the body. The lungs shrink in proportion to the volume reduction of the gas phase. The alveolar membrane thickens in accordance with the collapse of the lungs, and the compressed air is driven into the rigid structures: the larger bronchi, the trachea, and the nasal cavity. Now, it has been observed in fin whales that the bony parts of the airways amounts to approximately one tenth of the lung volume.[7] Therefore, at 100 M. depths the lungs have collapsed and the initial volume of lung gas has been reduced to one tenth and is contained within the rigid dead space. The alveolar membrane has become greatly thickened during the process and very little gas can diffuse into the blood. When the animals swim towards the sur-

123

face, these processes are reversed and decompression illness is avoided.[7]

It may be said that the diving mammals are not in any danger of contracting the bends because they do not receive any supply of air at high pressure while submerged. However, it is well known that a series of repeated skin dives increases the possibility of decompression illness in humans. Moreover, the incidence of caisson disease due to accumulation of nitrogen increases with increasing amounts of body fat since the fats are very good nitrogen solvents. For these reasons, diving mammals might well incur decompression illness were it not for the protective mechanisms discussed above.

REFERENCES

1. Andersen, H. T.: Physiological adaptations in diving vertebrates, Physiol. Rev. **46**:212, 1966.
2. Kooyman, G. L.: Maximum diving capacities of the Weddell seal, Leptonychotes weddelli, Science **151**:1553, 1966.
3. Heezen, B. C.: Whales entangled in deep sea cables, Deep-sea Res. **4**:105, 1957.
4. Kooyman, G. L., and Andersen, H. T.: Deep diving, *in* Andersen, H. T., editor: The biology of marine mammals, New York, Academic Press, Inc. In preparation.
5. Bohr, C.: Bidrag til svømmefuglernes fysiologi (In Danish), K. Danske Vidensk. Selsk. no. 2, 1897.
6. Dill, D. B., and Edwards, H. T.: Respiration and metabolism in a young crocodile (Crocodylus acutus, Cuvier), Copeia **1**:1931.
7. Scholander, P. F.: Experimental investigations on the respiratory function in diving mammals and birds, Hvalrådets Skrifter no. 22. Norske Videnskaps-Akad., Oslo 1940.
8. Scholander, P. F., Irving, L., and Grinnell, S. W.: On the temperature and metabolism of the seal during diving, J. Cell. & Comp. Physiol. **19**:67, 1942.
9. Irving, L.: On the ability of warm-blooded animals to survive without breathing, Scient. Monthly, New York **38**:422, 1934.
10. Bert, P.: Leçons sur la physiologie comparée de la respiration, Paris, 1870, Baillière, pp. 526–553.
11. Richet, C.: De la résistance des canards à l'asphyxie, J. Physiol. Pathol. gén. **1**:641, 1898.
12. Andersen, H. T.: Physiological adjustments to prolonged diving in the American alligator, Alligator mississippiensis, Acta physiol., Scandinav. **53**:23, 1961.
13. Artom, C.: Sur les rapports entre le rhythme de la respiration et le rythme du coeur chez les oiseaux, Arch. Néerl. Physiol. **10**:376, 1926.
14. Harrison, R. J., and Tomlinson, J. W. D.: Normal and experimental diving in the common seal (Phoca vitulina), Extr. Mam. **24**:386, 1960.
15. Lombroso, U.: Über die reflexhemmung des herzens während der reflektorischen atmungshemmung bei verschiedenen tieren, Ztschr. Biol. **61**:517, 1913.
16. Murdaugh, H. V., Jr., Seabury, J. C., and Mitchell, W. L.: Electrocardiogram of the diving seal, Circulation Res. **9**:358, 1961.
17. Andersen, H. T.: Hyperpotassemia and electrocardiographic changes in the duck during prolonged diving, Acta physiol. Scandinav. **63**:292, 1965.
18. Irving, L., Scholander, P. F., and Grinnell, S. W.: The regulation of arterial blood pressure in the seal during diving, Am. J. Physiol. **135**:557, 1942.
19. Hollenberg, N. K., and Uvnäs, B.: The role of the cardiovascular response in the resistance to asphyxia of avian divers, Acta physiol. Scandinav. **58**:150, 1963.
20. Murdaugh, H. V., Jr., Schmidt-Nielsen, B., Wood, J. W., and Mitchell, W. L.: Cessation of renal function during diving in the trained seal (Phoca vitulina), J. Cell. & Comp. Physiol. **58**:261, 1961.
21. Sykes, A. H.: Submersion anuria in the duck, J. Physiol. (Lond.) **184**:16 P, 1966.
22. Elsner, R., Franklin, D. L., van Citters, R. L., and Kenney, D. W.: Cardiovascular defense against asphyxia, Science **153**:941, 1966.
23. Scholander, P. F.: Physiological adaptations to diving in animals and man, Harvey Lect. **57**:93, 1961–62.
24. Scholander, P. F.: Animals in aquatic environments: Diving mammals and birds, *in* Handbook of physiology, Sec. IV, Adaptations to the environment, Washington, D. C., 1964, Am. Physiol. Soc., pp. 729–739.
25. Irving, L.: Comparative anatomy and physiology of gas transport mechanisms, *in* Handbook of physiology, Sec. III, Respiration, Washington, D. C., 1964, Am. Physiol. Soc., vol. 1, pp. 198–209.
26. Irving, L., Scholander, P. F., and Grinnell, S. W.: The respiration of the porpoise, Tursiops truncatus, J. Cell. & Comp. Physiol. **17**:145, 1941.

Advances in Decompression Research

H. R. SCHREINER, Ph.D.

The toxicity of oxygen at high partial pressures makes it mandatory that an inert diluent be used to supply the diver at depth with oxygen at a physiologically acceptable partial pressure. Unless the use of liquids becomes practical, there is no alternative to the use of inert gases for this purpose.

Biological systems take up inert gases when exposed to them under pressure. The reduction of this pressure, that is, the process of decompression is the subject of this discussion. Decompression represents one of the key problems facing man-in-the-sea. This is so because the gases that are taken up by the body tissues during the high pressure phase of a dive must be allowed to leave the body during ascent to the surface in a manner which precludes the formation of bubbles, or if bubbles do form, prevents their growth to a size that can inflict damage to the diver.

Our knowledge of the factors that must be considered in making decompression procedures safe today, some 60 years after Haldane's[1] pioneering work, is still very limited. The consequences of this relative ignorance are compounded by the rapid increase in depths to which man is today diving to seek information or to provide services. Those who are charged with devising means for the return of man from such deep dives know very well how frustratingly slow the rate of decompression research is and how inadequate the current level of its private and public support. Nevertheless, significant advances have been made in this field, and we need to consider some of them.

It is possible to discern three broad aspects of decompression research. These are: the transport of inert gases in the body, gas phase separation and the growth of bubbles, and the pathophysiology of decompression sickness. This report will deal largely with the gas transport aspect of decompression research. My colleagues at this Symposium will devote their attention primarily to the remaining two topics.

Specifically, we should like to review some of the current attempts to obtain, by the preferential, sequential or simultaneous use of different inert gases, indications of a significant decompression advantage to the diver or, for that matter, to the astronaut exposed to a two-gas spacecabin atmosphere. If one considers that decompression from a two-hour dive to 1,000 feet takes on the order of two to three days,[2] even if all goes well, and that similar dives to 2,000 or 3,000 feet will generate decompression obligations that may take weeks to satisfy by current techniques, it then becomes clear that without radical improvements in decompression procedures such dives, although probably feasible, would require a level of financial and personnel support so exorbitant that their conduct for commercial purposes will hardly be practical.[3]

To provide a rational basis for the development of improved breathing gas mixtures for divers (and astronauts) it is necessary to consider, first, the factors that govern the uptake of inert gases by and their elimination from the body, and then to gain some insight into the conditions which determine whether gas bubbles will form and grow in the tissues during and after decompression.

On the basis of the classical work of Jones,[4] one is obliged to consider that tissue perfusion with blood, rather than the diffusion properties of inert gases, govern the rate of uptake and elimination (Fig. 1). If we make the reasonable assumption that blood entering the lungs becomes completely equilibrated with inert gas, then the quantity of inert gas entering the arterial circulation per unit of time is given as the product of perfusion rate $\dot{Q}$, coefficient α of inert gas solubility in blood and the alveolar partial pressure P of the inert gas. The quantity of inert gas leaving a given tissue per unit of time in turn is given by the product of perfusion rate $\dot{Q}$, coefficient α of inert gas solubility in blood and π, the partial pressure of the inert gas dissolved in the tissue.

The difference between these two quantities of gas clearly represents the amount of gas added to or taken away from the tissue per time unit. This relationship can be expressed as a differential equation which states that the rate of change of inert gas partial pressure dissolved in a tissue is, at all times, proportional to the difference between alveolar and tissue inert gas partial pressure. The proportionally constant k is the specific time constant of inert gas transport and is equal to the product of perfusion rate $\dot{Q}$ and the coefficient of partition of the inert gas between blood and tissue. This gas transport equation (Fig. 2) can be integrated and numerically solved when the rate of change of the alveolar inert gas pressure, P, is a constant. With a knowledge of the initial values of P and π it is, therefore, possible to compute the inert gas partial pressure π at any time during linear or stepwise ascent or descent for any tissue for which the value of k can be determined or

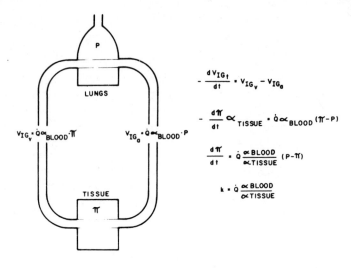

Fig. 1. Schematic representation of perfusion-limited inert gas transport between the lungs and peripheral tissue.

GAS TRANSPORT EQUATION:

$$\frac{d\pi}{dt} = k\,(P-\pi)$$

GENERAL SOLUTION:

$$\pi = e^{-\int k\,dt}\left[\int Pe^{\int k\,dt}\,dt\right] + c_1 e^{-\int k\,dt}$$

SPECIAL SOLUTION FOR $\dfrac{dP}{dt} = C$:

$$\pi = P_0 + C\left(t - \frac{1}{k}\right) - \left(P_0 - \pi_0 - \frac{C}{k}\right)e^{-kt}$$

$$k = \dot{Q}\,\frac{\propto BLOOD}{\propto TISSUE}$$

Fig. 2.

deduced from its perfusion and fat content.[5]

In order to avoid the formation of gas bubbles in the tissues, the value of π, which is the inert gas tension in a given tissue, must not be allowed to exceed an empirically determined value which varies apparently with depth and specific time constant k of inert gas transport. This value is considered to be the maximum tissue inert gas tension associated with a still acceptable risk of phase separation.[6,7] It is possible, by the way, to decompress a diver without sustaining any supersaturation in his tissues if the time required for decompression is not of great concern. The isobaric, or oxygen window, principle of decompression which makes this possible was developed by Behnke[8] (Fig. 3) and takes advantage, primarily, of the arteriovenous difference in P_{O_2}. By reducing the ambient pressure, P_A, in such a way that it always equals the dissolved inert gas pressure π in the tissue, it is possible to produce an outward flow of inert gases which is proportional to the sum of arterial oxygen, carbon dioxide and water vapor tensions. While unquestionably a safe technique, Buckles[9] has calculated that decompression after a one hour dive to 300 feet would require 70 hours by the oxygen window technique, as compared to ten hours for conventional decompression involving supersaturation. Because of this time penalty, decompression schedules based on permissible levels of supersaturation will be more attractive in most instances. We shall, therefore, return now to our consideration of the perfusion-limited model of inert gas transport and the manner in which it is employed in dealing with different inert gases.

If we assume that tissue consists of a variable mixture of fat and water (Fig. 4) and further assume that the solubility of inert gases in blood is equal to that in water, the specific time constant k (or half-time of gas transport $t_{\frac{1}{2}}$) of a particular inert gas can be derived from the relative solubility of an inert gas in fat and water and from the fat fraction X of a given tissue, as long as the rate of tissue perfusion is known. The basic gas transport equation can, therefore, be rewritten as shown in Fig. 5.

Although we lack accurate numerical data, certain limits can be set for the rate of perfusion and the fat fraction of a tissue. The distribution coefficient of an inert gas between fat and water is generally known with precision. In the development of our mathematical description of inert gas transport, we have deliberately assumed that the rate of perfusion in man ranges from a minimum of 0.0085 min^{-1} to a maximum which is greater than 0.3 min^{-1}, and that the fat fraction X of human tissue may range from

129

$$\frac{d\pi}{dt} = -k\,(\pi - P)$$

AMBIENT GAS PRESSURE $\quad P_A = P + P_{AO_2} + P_{ACO_2} + P_{H_2O}$

TISSUE GAS PRESSURE $\quad P_T = \pi + P_{VO_2} + P_{VCO_2} + P_{H_2O}$

$$\underline{IF\ P_A = P_T:}$$

$$\pi - P = P_{AO_2} - P_{VO_2} + P_{ACO_2} - P_{VCO_2}$$

$$\underline{IF\ \pi = P_A:}$$

$$\pi - P = P_{AO_2} + P_{ACO_2} + P_{H_2O}$$

Fig. 3. The isobaric (oxygen window) principle of decompression. (Ref. Behnke[8]).

$$k = \dot{Q}\;\frac{\alpha\ BLOOD}{\alpha\ TISSUE}$$

$$k \cong \dot{Q}\;\frac{\alpha\ WATER}{(1-X)\alpha\ WATER + X\,\alpha\ FAT}$$

$$k \cong \dot{Q}\;\frac{1}{1 + X\left(\dfrac{\alpha\ FAT}{\alpha\ WATER} - 1\right)}$$

$$\frac{\alpha\ FAT}{\alpha\ WATER}:\quad HELIUM : 1.7 \qquad NEON : 2.1$$
$$NITROGEN : 5.1 \qquad ARGON : 5.3$$

$$k = \frac{\ell n\,2}{t\,\frac{1}{2}}$$

Fig. 4.

0 to 1.0.[10] For the purpose of following the time course of inert gas partial pressures dissolved in various gas exchange units of the human body, let us consider the combination of a few representative values of $\dot{Q}$ and X. The mathematical model of inert gas transport in use in our laboratory employs 15 such combinations, as outlined in Table I. Displayed

130

$$\frac{d\Pi}{dt} = \frac{\dot{Q}(P-\Pi)}{1+X\left(\dfrac{\alpha\ FAT}{\alpha\ WATER} - 1\right)}$$

Fig. 5. Gas transport equation.

TABLE I

HALF-TIMES OF INERT GAS TRANSPORT

BLOOD FLOW $\dot{Q}$ (CC/MIN/CC)	PERCENT FAT CONTENT OF TISSUE			
	0	30	70	100
0.3	$\frac{He\ \vert\ Ne}{N_2\ \vert\ A_R}$	$\frac{3\ \vert\ 3}{5\ \vert\ 5}$	$\frac{3\ \vert\ 4}{9\ \vert\ 9}$	$\frac{4\ \vert\ 5}{12\ \vert\ 12}$
0.1	$\frac{7\ \vert\ 7}{7\ \vert\ 7}$	$\frac{8\ \vert\ 9}{15\ \vert\ 16}$	$\frac{10\ \vert\ 12}{27\ \vert\ 28}$	$\frac{12\ \vert\ 15}{35\ \vert\ 37}$
0.03	$\frac{23\ \vert\ 23}{23\ \vert\ 23}$	$\frac{28\ \vert\ 31}{52\ \vert\ 53}$	$\frac{34\ \vert\ 41}{89\ \vert\ 93}$	$\frac{39\ \vert\ 49}{118\ \vert\ 122}$
0.0085	$\frac{81\ \vert\ 81}{81\ \vert\ 81}$	$\frac{99\ \vert\ 108}{182\ \vert\ 187}$	$\frac{122\ \vert\ 145}{315\ \vert\ 327}$	$\frac{139\ \vert\ 171}{416\ \vert\ 432}$

here are the calculated half-times, in minutes, of the transport of helium, neon, nitrogen and argon for combinations of four representative rates of blood blood flow and four levels of tissue fat content. Even though each particular combination of blood flow and tissue fat content defines a gas exchange "compartment" in the anatomic sense, we must keep in mind that a given gas transport half-time does not necessarily correspond to an anatomic entity, since various combinations of blood flow $\dot{Q}$ and partition coefficient $\dfrac{\alpha\ \text{blood}}{\alpha\ \text{tissue}}$ can (as we have seen in Fig. 2) give rise to one and the same value of k, and hence, $t_{\frac{1}{2}}$.

This view of inert gas transport, although not new,[11] is by no means generally accepted, as we shall see later on. It does, however, provide a rational base that is required for the interpretation of experimental decompression studies of different inert gases. [12-19]

TABLE II

Score	Symptoms of Decompression Sickness*
0	None
1	Indefinite and Transient
2	Mild Disturbances in Walking
3	Dragging of Hind Limb(s)
4	Paralysis of Hind Quarters
5	Paralysis of Front and Hind Quarters
6	Death

*(Ref. Philp and Gowdey[20]).

TABLE III

STAGE DECOMPRESSION TO 510 MM HG FOLLOWING
TWO HOUR EXPOSURES TO 4650 MM HG*

Inert Gas	Mean Bends Score For Sprague-Dawley Rats %		% Severe Bends
Helium	21/96	(22)	19
Neon	13/90	(14)	13
Nitrogen	134/144	(93)	96
(Oxygen Concentration at Maximum Pressure = 20%)			

*(Ref. Doebbler at el.[14]).

The amount of gas present in solution in a given gas transport compartment in relation to the total pressure is believed to be an important predictor of decompression sickness. The higher the ratio of dissolved inert gas pressure to total pressure, the greater is the probability that gas bubbles will form. Known as the Haldane Ratio, the value of this parameter on reaching sea level (or, generally speaking, a target baseline total pressure) is termed "surfacing ratio," a term of which we shall make extensive use in this discussion later on.

Small animals such as rats are quite useful for basic orientation studies in decompression research, even though they do not approximate man in terms of size, shape, or perfusion characteristics. The now classic method of Philp and Gowdey[20] permits a fairly objective assessment of decompression damage in rats and guinea pigs' by scoring their response during a post-decompression observation period while being forced to walk slowly. This arbitrary scoring system is shown in Table II.

By adding the individual bends scores, an integral bends score can be obtained for a group of animals. By dividing this integral bends score by the maximum bends score attainable (total number of animals x 6), a mean bends score (MBS) is derived which represents a numerical measure (ranging from 0 to 1) of the relative degree of failure of a given compression-decompression regime.

Doebbler and associates,[14] at our Laboratory, employed this approach to determine the effects of helium, neon, argon and nitrogen on the relative susceptibility of Sprague-Dawley rats and guinea pigs to decompression sickness. Using female animals of carefully matched weight, they observed the mean bends scores (Table III) after stage decompression following two hours of exposure to 80-20 mixtures of helium, neon or nitrogen with oxygen at a pressure equivalent to 178 feet of seawater. These results might be interpreted as suggesting that neon exhibits a decompression advantage over helium, but show clearly for both these gases an advantage over nitrogen.

Now, using data from this same experiment, we have computed the surfacing ratios (i.e., sum of inert gas partial pressures divided by total pressure) for the 15 compartments of our gas transport model for the three inert gases examined. Inspection of this data (Fig. 6) shows that the surfacing ratio at the end of the stage decompression was for the nitrogen exposures highest in the well-perfused tissues (Compartments 1–7); for the helium-exposed animals this ratio was highest in the poorly perfused tissues (Compartments 8–15). If surfacing ratio, without regard to the nature of the gas, and the half-time of the tissue is the chief factor which determines the outcome of decompression, then the experimental results (Relative MBS; He: Ne: N_2 = 0.22: 0.14: 0: 93) would lead one to believe that the poorly perfused tissues represented by Compartments 8–15 are of no importance in the decompression of small animals. This assumption is not entirely correct, however, since experience has shown[6,7] that slow gas exchange compartments will produce bends with a smaller surfacing ratio than can be sustained by rapidly clearing tissues.

The surfacing ratios for neon-exposed animals are slightly larger than for helium-exposed rats in the well-perfused compartments, and should, therefore, be associated with a higher, and not a lower, mean

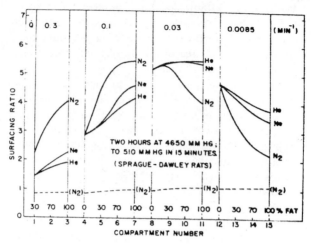

Fig. 6. *Computed surfacing ratios of dissolved inert gases in 15 perfusion-limited tissue compartments.*

TABLE IV

RAPID DECOMPRESSION TO 510 MM HG FOLLOWING
TWO HOUR EXPOSURES TO 4650 MM HG*

Inert Gas	Mean Bends Score For Sprague-Dawley Rats %		% Severe Bends
Helium	27/48	(56)	50
Neon	26/48	(54)	50

(Oxygen Concentration at Maximum Pressure = 20%)

(Ref. Doebbler et al.[14]).

bends score than that produced by helium. Considering the rapidity of clearance of both helium and neon from the well-perfused tissues of the animal, it is not unreasonable to assume that for these gases the less well-perfused tissues (Compartments 8–15) assume critical importance, and in these compartments the surfacing ratio in the helium-exposed rats actually exceeds the surfacing ratio calculated for the neon-exposed rats. This would provide a satisfactory explanation for the observed slight decompression advantage of neon.

In another experiment we attempted to differentiate between the effects of helium and neon during the rapid decompression of rats (Table IV). This failed to demonstrate the decompression advantage of neon that was seen after stage decompression.

134

Although the calculated surfacing ratios after rapid decompression (Fig. 7) are qualitatively similar to those obtained after stage decompression, any possible decompression advantage of neon in the slowly perfused tissues may have been obliterated by the generally higher surfacing ratios sustained in this experiment which may have produced massive bubble formation irrespective of the nature of the inert gas present.

I should like to draw your attention to the fact

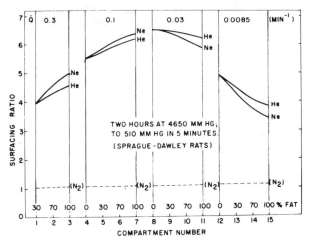

Fig. 7. *Computed surfacing ratios of dissolved inert gases in 15 perfusion-limited tissue compartments.*

TABLE V

RAPID DECOMPRESSION TO 100 MM HG FOLLOWING
SATURATION EXPOSURES TO 756 MM HG*

Inert Gas	Mean Bends Score For Sprague-Dawley Rats %		% Severe Bends
Helium	12/36	(33)	0
Neon	13/36	(36)	17
Nitrogen	33/72	(46)	42
Argon	27/36	(75)	100

(Oxygen Concentration at Maximum Pressure = 20%)

*(*Ref. Hamilton et al.*[3]).

that after exposure to helium or neon, the tissues of these experimental animals still contained nitrogen at a substantial partial pressure, which is shown by the

135

dashed lines in Figs. 6 and 7. We are, therefore, not really comparing neon vs. helium here, but a neon-nitrogen mixture with a helium-nitrogen mixture. This must be kept in mind in interpreting the results of inert gas decompression studies in which the indigenous tissue nitrogen was not completely removed prior to the decompression experience.

To date the only experiment in which this was done was performed by Hamilton and his associates,[17] at our Laboratory (Table V). Male, obese Sprague-Dawley rats were exposed to mixtures of oxygen and helium, neon, nitrogen or argon for 48 hours at ground level before they were rapidly decompressed to the equivalent altitude of 47,000 feet while breathing oxygen. Under these circumstances of decompression after a saturation exposure, the surfacing ratios in all compartments decreased in the order of argon-nitrogen-neon-helium, and the mean bends score paralleled these surfacing ratios, which are graphically displayed in Fig. 8. Up to this point, then, the experimental evidence examined so far

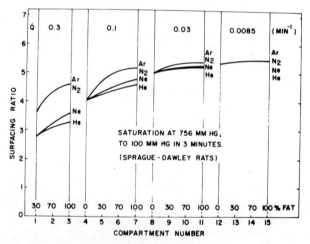

Fig. 8. Computed surfacing ratios of dissolved inert gases in 15 perfusion-limited tissue compartments.

can be explained on the basis of differences in surfacing ratios, with the proviso that gases with a low solubility fat-water ratio may leave the well-perfused tissues so rapidly that the occurrence of a phase separation may hinge upon the magnitude of the

TABLE VI

RAPID DECOMPRESSION TO 510 MM HG FOLLOWING
TWO HOUR EXPOSURES TO 4650 MM HG*

Inert Gas	Mean Bends Score For Guinea Pigs %		% Severe Bends
Nitrogen	41/48	(85)	100
Argon	48/48	(100)	100

(Oxygen Concentration at Maximum Pressure = 20%)

*(Ref. Doebbler et al.[14]).

TABLE VII

RAPID DECOMPRESSION TO 760 MM HG FOLLOWING
ONE HOUR EXPOSURES TO 7370 MM HG*

Inert Gas	Mean Bends Score For Wistar Rats %		% Severe Bends
Helium	122/360	(34)	45
Helium-Neon (30:70)	98/240	(41)	50
Helium-Neon (50:50)	38/120	(32)	40
Nitrogen	130/240	(54)	57
Argon	120/120	(100)	100

(Oxygen Concentration at Maximum Pressure = 20%)

*(Ref. Bennett et al.[13]).

surfacing ratio in the less-well-perfused tissues.

Nitrogen and argon have almost identical transport characteristics and should, if surfacing ratios were the sole factor governing decompression success, produce identical results. Hamilton's data (Table V) clearly show that this is not the case; Doebbler and his associates[14] corroborated this finding, using guinea pigs (Table VI). The surfacing ratios computed for this experiment are shown in Fig. 9.

Similar observations have been made with Wistar rats by Bennett and co-workers (Table VII). By assigning a score of four to spinal bends and a score of six to animals that died following decompression from a one-hour exposure to a pressure equivalent to 290 feet of seawater, results reported by these investigators were converted to the mean bends scores displayed in Table VII for comparison purposes. An interesting observation made in the course of this study is the low mean bends score obtained with a 50:50 mixture of neon and helium. This score is

137

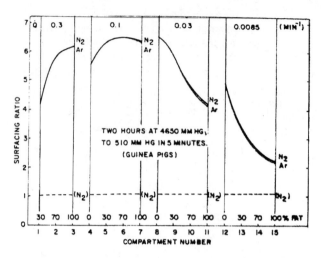

Fig. 9. *Computed surfacing ratios of dissolved inert gases in 15 perfusion-limited tissue compartments.*

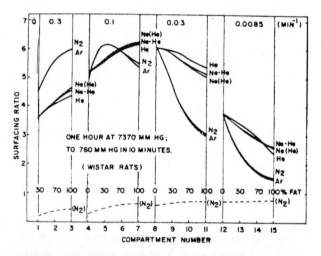

Fig. 10. *Computed surfacing ratios of dissolved inert gases in 15 perfusion-limited tissue compartments.*

slightly lower than that obtained for helium alone, or for crude neon which contains close to 30% helium. A review of the calculated surfacing ratios for this series (Fig. 10) provides no basis for an

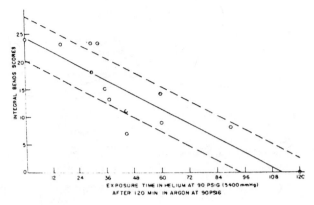

Fig. 11. *Integral bends scores of Sprague-Dawley rats as a function of time of exposure to helium-oxygen after two hours under argon-oxygen. (Solid line represents averaged response, broken line denote ±one standard deviation.*

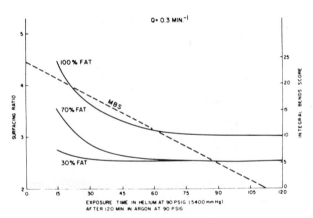

Fig. 12. *Computed surfacing ratios of total dissolved inert gas in three tissue compartments (30, 70 and 100% fat) perfused at the rate of 0.3 cc/min/cc.[9]*

explanation of this particular result, and makes it clear, as did the comparison between nitrogen and argon, that surfacing ratios by and in themselves do not determine, even within a particular compartment, the success of decompression.

This has been most tellingly demonstrated by Doebbler and his coworkers,[15] who determined the mean bends score of animals that had been exposed to an oxygen-argon mixture at 5,400 mm. Hg (202 feet of seawater) for two hours, followed by addi-

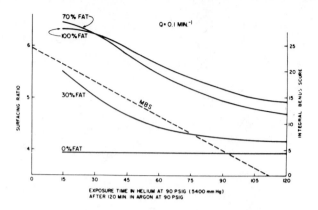

Fig. 13. Computed surfacing ratios of total dissolved inert gas in four tissue compartments (0, 30, 70 and 100% fat) perfused at the rate of 0.1 cc/min/cc.[9]

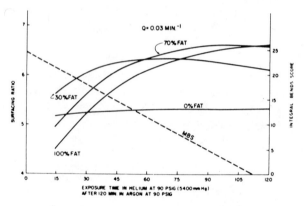

Fig. 14. Computed surfacing ratios of total dissolved inert gas in four tissue compartments (0, 30, 70 and 100% fat) perfused at the rate of 0.03 cc/min/cc.[9]

tional exposures at that depth to an oxygen-helium mixture. Fig. 11 shows how in this experiment the integral bends score decreases approximately linearly, from a maximum of 24, or 100% fatalities, with the additional time the animals spent at 5,400 mm. Hg breathing oxygen-helium.

Figs. 12 and 13 show that the surfacing ratios of the well-perfused tissues, especially those containing significant amounts of fat, actually increased during the period immediately following the shift from argon to helium at depth, reflecting the fact that in these tissues helium was taken up at a rate exceeding that

140

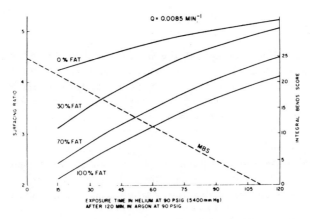

Fig. 15. Computed surfacing ratios of total dissolved inert gas in four tissue compartments (0, 30, 70 and 100% fat) perfused at the rate of 0.0085 cc/min/cc.[9]

of the removal of argon. It is, therefore, clear that a fundamental difference exists between helium and argon in the manner in which these gases affect the outcome of decompression, and that this difference is not merely a function of the surfacing ratio. If tissues perfused at a rate of 0.03–0.0085 min.$^{-1}$ actually exist in the rat, this interpretation of the present experiment becomes even more convincing, because in these poorly perfused tissues (Figs. 14 and 15), the surfacing ratio continues to increase as the mean bends score decreases.

From this body of preliminary experimental evidence, we can draw the following corollaries:

1. Surfacing ratios reflect the relative decompression advantage of various inert gases only after a saturation exposure.

2. When the exposure to a given inert gas is short of saturation, the significance of the surfacing ratio as a determinator of decompression success must be modified by considering the rate of perfusion of the compartments in which supersaturation exists, and the nature of the inert gas breathed.

3. When two gases produce identical, or near-identical, surfacing ratios, the injury produced by the more soluble gas

141

will be greater than that caused by the less soluble gas.

This appraisal of the experimental evidence on hand would not be complete without a critique of the assumptions that are inherent in the perfusion-limited view of gas transport which we have used to interpret it. This view, which is shared by many workers[7,21-23] in the field, is based upon the assumption that the diffusion coefficients of inert gases in cytoplasm are of the same order of magnitude as those determined in water or extracellular fluid. This assumption has been challenged by Hills,[24] who points out that when diffusion coefficients for cellular materials are determined by truly transient methods, they turn out to be smaller by factors of 10^2–10^4 than diffusion coefficients estimated by steady-state techniques. These techniques assume tissue to be a homogenous diffusion medium and, therefore, do not distinguish between solute molecules which bypass cells by preferential diffusion through extracellular fluid and those which migrate through the cytoplasm.

The more or less conventional view that limited supersaturation of inert gas may exist in the tissues is also challenged by Hills, [25-27] who argues on thermodynamic grounds that phase separation should occur whenever there is supersaturation. It is difficult to interpret experimental data from Hills' point of view since his concept of gas transport is not readily subject to mathematical treatment. It relies importantly on thermal and pneumatic analogs which represent the radial diffusion of inert gas from a cylindrical capillary into the surrounding cytoplasm. In this postulated model all gas in excess of equilibrium at any point in the cytoplasm will separate from solution at that point. If this view is correct then hydrogen, which diffuses faster than any

TABLE VIII

INERT GAS SOLUBILITIES

| Gas | CC STP/1000 Gm. Solvent | | |
	Water	Fat	Fat/Water
Hydrogen	16	50	3.1
Helium	8	15	1.7
Neon	10	19	2.1
Nitrogen	13	67	5.1
Argon	28	140	5.3

other inert gas, should permit the most rapid ascent from depth consistent with safety. If, on the other hand, the perfusion-limited model provides a more nearly correct description of inert gas transport in the body, then hydrogen, which resembles nitrogen and argon in its absolute and relative fat and water solubility (Table VIII) more than it resembles helium or neon, should resemble these gases also in its effect on decompression success. This critical experiment remains to be carried out.

References

1. BOYCOTT, A. W.; DAMANT, G. C.; and HALDANE, J. S.: Prevention of Compressed Air Illness. *J Hyg* (London), 8:342–443, 1908.
2. BUEHLMANN, A. A.: Personal communication, 1967.
3. HAMILTON, R. W., JR. and SCHREINER, H. R.: Putting and Keeping Man in the Sea. *Chem Eng*, 75:263–270, 1968.
4. JONES, H. B.: Respiratory System: Nitrogen Elimination. (Ed. Glasser, O.). *Med Phy*, 2:855–871, 1950.
5. SCHREINER, H. R. and KELLEY, P. L.: Computation Methods for Decompression from Deep Divers. Proceedings Third Symposium Underwater Physiology. (Ed. Lambertsen, C. J. *Williams & Wilkins*, Baltimore, 1967.
6. SCHREINER, H. R.: Mathematical Approaches to Decompression. *Internat J Biometerol*, 11:301–310, 1967.
7. WORKMAN, R. D.: Caclulation of Decompression Schedules for Nitrogen-Oxygen and Helium-Oxygen Dives. *Res Report* 6–65. U. S. Navy Experimental Diving Unit, Washington D. C. 1965.
8. BEHNKE, A. R.: Medical Aspects of Work in Pressurized Tunnel Operations. *Transit Insurance Admin*, San Francisco, Calif., 1968.
9. BUCKLES, R. G.: Etiology of Decompression Sickness: Characteristics of Bubble Formation, *in vivo*. *Research Report No.* 1(*AD* 661841) Bethesda, Md. Naval Medical Research Institute, 1967.
10. SCHREINER, H. R.: Safe Ascent After Deep Dives. *Rev Subaqu Physiol Hyperbar Med*, (Paris), 1:28–37, 1968.
11. BJURSTEDT, H. and SEVERIN, G.: The Prevention of Decompression Sickness and Nitrogen Narcosis by the Use of Hydrogen as a Substitute of Nitrogen. (The Arne Zetterstrom Method of Deep Sea Diving). *Mil Surg*, 103:107–116, 1948.
12. BEARD, S. E.; ALLEN, T. H.; MCIVER, R. G. and BANCROFT, R. W.: Comparison of Helium and Nitrogen in Production of Bends in Simulated Orbital Flights. *Aerospace Med*, 38:331–337, 1967.
13. BENNETT, P. B. and HAYWARD, A. J.: Relative Decompression Sickness Hazards in Rats of Neon and Other Inert Gases. *Aerospace Med*, 39:301–302, 1968.

14. DOEBBLER, G. F.; BUCHHEIT, R. G. and SCHREINER, H. R.: Effect of Helium, Neon, Nitrogen, and Argon on the Relative Susceptibility of Animals to Depth Decompression Sickness. 38th Annual Meeting, *Aerospace Med Assn*, Washington, D.C., April 12, 1967.

15. DOEBBLER, G. F.; BUCHHEIT, R. G.; and SCHREINER, H. R.: Unpublished Data.

16. GERSH, I.; HAWKINSON, G. E.; and JENNEY, E. H.: Comparison of Vascular and Extravascular Bubbles Following Decompression from High Pressure Atmospheres of Oxygen, Helium-Oxygen, Argon-Oxygen and Air. *J Cell Comp Physiol*, 26:63–74, 1945.

17. HAMILTON, R. W., JR. and SCHREINER, H. R.: Effects of Helium, Neon, Nitrogen and Argon on the Relative Susceptibility of Animals to Altitude Decompression Sickness. 38th Annual Meeting, *Aerospace Med Assn*, Washington, D.C., April 11, 1967.

18. HELLER, H. and BUEHLMANN, A. A.: Deep Diving and Short Decompression by Breathing Mixed Gases. *J Appl Physiol*, 20:1267–1270, 1965.

19. SMITH, E. B.: Decompression Experiments with Various Gases. Proceedings Third Symposium, Underwater Physiology. Lambertsen, C. J. Ed. *Williams & Wilkins*, Baltimore, 1967.

20. PHILP, R. B. and GOWDEY, C. W.: Decompression Sickness in Rats During Exercise at Simulated Altitudes After Exposure to Compressed Air. Aerospace Med, •33:1433–1437, 1962.

21. GORANSSON, A.; LUNDGREN, C.; and LUNDIN, G.: A Theoretical Model for the Computation of Decompression Tables for Divers. *Nature*, 199:384–385, 1963.

22. Lundgren, C. E. G.: Experimental Decompression Sickness in Goats in Relation to Predicted Tissue Gas Supersaturation. *Forsarmed*, 3:Suppl. 3, 1967.

23. RUFF, S.: Theoretische Untersuchungen zur Entstehung von Gasembolien und Gasblasen im Gewebe. *Der Anaes*, 15:317–319, 1966.

24. HILLS, B. A.: A Thermodynamic and Kinetic Approach to Decompression Sickness. *Libraries Board of South Australia*, Adelaide, 1966.

25. HILLS, B. A.: A Pneumatic Analogue for Predicting the Occurrence of Decompression Sickness. *Med Biol Eng*, 5:421–432, 1967.

26. HILLS, B. A.: A Thermal Analogue for the Optimal Decompression of Divers: Theory. *Physics Med Biol*, 12:437–444, 1967.

27. HILLS, B. A.: A Thermal Analogue for the Optimal Decompression of Divers: Construction and Use. *Physics Med Biol*, 12:445–454, 1967.

144

THE POSSIBLE EFFECT ON ATHLETIC PERFORMANCES OF MEXICO CITY'S ALTITUDE

W. P. LEARY AND C. H. WYNDHAM

Wyndham *et al.*, in 1963,[1] and Leary and Wyndham in 1965,[2] presented the results of their studies on the pulmonary ventilations and maximum oxygen intakes of fit young men and international class athletes, respectively, while they exercised in Johannesburg, which lies at what is classed as a medium altitude, i.e. 5,780 feet above sea-level. These studies showed that pulmonary ventilation is markedly increased during exercise at this altitude compared with sea-level values and, in consequence, maximum oxygen intakes are reduced.

As a complementary study, the performances of South African athletes at sea-level and at medium altitudes have been analysed, to see whether there is any support in the recorded performances, for the deleterious effects of medium altitude.

In South Africa competitive athletics is largely confined to the urban areas, particularly Durban, Cape Town and Port Elizabeth which are coastal centres, and (inland high-veld centres) Johannesburg, Pretoria and Bloemfontein. The majority of important track meetings take place at altitudes of 4,000 feet or above and since 1952 the national championship meeting has been held at sea-level only 3 times.

The results of this analysis are of more than merely national interest. The next Olympic Games are due to be held in Mexico City, which lies at an altitude of 7,000 feet above sea-level. It is realized that the performances of the athletes may be affected deleteriously and that there may be even some danger to unacclimatized men. Precise information is lacking on the extent of deterioration in performance that can be expected at the altitude of Mexico City. This analysis gives some indication of the extent to which this might happen.

Considerable interest is being shown in this subject in international athletic circles. Physiological studies are being carried out by national research bodies on British, Swedish, American and Japanese athletes in Mexico City and an International Symposium was held recently at Magglinen, in Switzerland, to discuss the physiological implication of athletics at medium altitudes to which this laboratory contributed.

ANALYSIS OF RECORDS

The data set out in Tables I - III are from statistics to be found in the *South African Athletics Annual* of 1964.

TABLE I. BEST PERFORMANCES RECORDED 1900–1964

Distance	Number of performances	Sea-level	3,500–5,000 ft.	Above 5,000 ft.
100 yards	48	3	33	12
440 yards	52	8	29	15
880 yards	53	21	25	7
1 mile	51	33	13	5
2 miles	52	34	10	8
3 miles	50	27	19	4
6 miles	50	29	11	10
Marathon	20	17	2	1

From Table I it is clear that the best performances recorded in the middle and long-distance events were at the coast. Sprinters have fared better at medium altitude.

TABLE II. WINNERS OF NATIONAL TRACK CHAMPIONSHIPS HELD AT 4,500 FT.

Year	Medal position	Domicile of winner			
		800 yards	1 mile	3 miles	6 miles
1955	Gold	Inland	Inland	Inland	Inland
	Silver	Coastal	Inland	Inland	Inland
	Bronze	Inland	Coastal	Inland	Inland
1958	Gold	Inland	Inland	Inland	Inland
	Silver	Inland	Inland	Inland	Coastal
	Bronze	Coastal	Inland	—	—
1963	Gold	Inland	Inland	Acclima-tized coastal	Inland
	Silver	Acclima-tized coastal	Acclima-tized coastal	Coastal	Inland
	Bronze	Coastal	Inland	Inland	Coastal

It is clear from Table II that South African championships held at medium altitude have been consistently dominated by athletes domiciled at such altitudes and those who acclimatized themselves by training at medium altitude for 3 - 4 weeks before the championship meeting.

146

Table III shows that the performances of a selection of international class athletes in the mile event have all been better by many seconds at sea-level.

TABLE III. DETERIORATION IN INDIVIDUAL PERFORMANCE AT 6,000 FT. ALTITUDE

Name	Year	Best coastal performance	Performance at 6,000 ft.
W. Lueg (Germany)	1955	4 min. 3 sec.	4 min. 20 sec·
G. Nielsen (Denmark)	1956	4 min. 1 sec.	4 min. 10 sec.
G. Pirie (UK)	1958	4 min. 3 sec.	4 min. 30 sec.
M. Halberg (NZ)	1958	3 min. 57·5 sec.	4 min. 8 sec.
D. Lamprecht (SA)	1965	3 min. 58 sec.	4 min. 8 sec.
Average		4 min. 0·5 sec.	4 min. 15·2 sec.

DISCUSSION

This analysis indicates that most of the best performances of middle and long-distance runners in South Africa in the last 60 years have been recorded at sea-level, whereas sprinters recorded better times at medium altitudes where the air density is less. Furthermore, the effect of acclimatization to altitude is shown in the fact that when the meeting took place at medium altitude nearly all of the best performances in middle-distance events were recorded by men who lived at these altitudes or by men who had travelled to and had trained at that altitude some weeks before the event.

The deterioration in performance of middle-distance runners at 6,000 feet is well shown in the poorer times of a group of international athletes in Johannesburg compared with the performances at sea-level.

It may be objected that athletic performances are dependent upon many other factors in addition to altitude. Such factors may include the conditions of the track, the wind velocity, the air temperature and humidity, etc. However, it is unlikely that any one of these factors would be consistently present in all of the medium altitude athletic meetings and not at sea-level.

From this analysis it appears that a number of conclusions could be drawn with reference to the performances of athletes in Mexico City. They are:

1. There is a consistent deterioration in performance (of coastal athletes) over middle and long-distance runs when these are held at medium altitude. Examination of Table III (and of data not set out here) shows that this deterioration ranges from 3% in the case of athletes who have undergone a 3 to 4-week period of training at medium altitude to more than 10% in those who are unacclimatized.

2. Medium altitude will not have any unfavourable effect on those running in the sprint events and, in fact, some small improvement may result.

3. It is to be expected that the middle and long-

147

distance events at Mexico City might well be dominated by relatively unknown athletes who are accustomed to living at medium altitudes and have made a successful adaptation to athletics at those altitudes.

4. Careful attention should be given by coaches to the proper acclimatization of athletes in the period before the Mexico City Olympic Games. A proper balance will have to be struck between the improved performances which occurs over a period of a few weeks and the eventual deterioration in performance which sets in if the period of acclimatization is prolonged too much.

To avoid these difficulties, athletic coaches will need to plan the training programme with the help of physiologists who have experience in exercise physiology.

This paper is published with the permission of the Transvaal and Orange Free State Chamber of Mines, Johannesburg.

REFERENCES

1. Wyndham. C. H., Strydom. N. B., Morrison, J., Peter, J., Williams, G., Bredell, G. A. G. and Joffe, A. (1963): J. Appl. Physiol., **18**, 361.
2. Leary, W. P. and Wyndham, C. H. (1965): S. Afr. Med. J., **39**, 651.

PHYSIOLOGICAL PROBLEMS EXPECTED AT THE MEXICO CITY OLYMPIC GAMES

C. H. WYNDHAM AND W. P. LEARY

There is a growing realization among medical men associated with athletics and other sports that the physical environment (comprising air temperature, relative humidity,
air movement and altitude above sea-level) in which
athletics events are carried out can affect performances
and even constitute a danger to life. Sir Adolphe
Abrahams[1] states that he knows of at least one death from
heat stroke in an athletic event on a very hot and humid
day. We have no doubt that if rectal temperatures were
measured immediately after sudden unexplained deaths in
sporting events, a much larger number of heat-stroke
deaths would have been shown. Recent reports in papers
on the deaths from heat stroke of young army recruits
carrying out exercises at a high level of work on very hot
days, lend support to this argument.

The next Olympic Games are due to be held in Mexico
City at an altitude of 7,000 feet above sea-level. There is
much concern in international athletic circles on the
possible effect that this altitude might have on the performances of the athletes and, also, as to whether there
might not be some danger to life. With these questions in
mind, a Symposium was held in December 1965 at
Magglinen in Switzerland on the 'Effects of medium altitude on athletic performances' to which exercise-physiolo-
gists, including those from this laboratory, were invited.

The altitude of Johannesburg is 5,780 feet (1,760 metres) and therefore a study of the physiology of exercise and of the performances of athletes at this altitude compared with sea-level will give some information on the limitations imposed on athletic performances by 'medium' altitudes.

In this paper is described the oxygen consumption/ventilation (BTPS) relationship during physical activities in Johannesburg and this relationship is compared with that obtaining at sea-level. The results are also given of studies of the maximum oxygen intakes and pulmonary ventilations of 10 national and international class athletes studied in Johannesburg and a comparison of these results is made with Astrand's observations on similar grade athletes studied at sea-level.[3]

The performances of sprinters and distance athletes at sea-level and at Johannesburg are compared in a separate paper.[6]

METHODS

The procedures used for the measurement of pulmonary ventilation and of maximum oxygen intake are described in detail in papers from this laboratory.[4,5,7] The subjects had physical characteristics as shown in Table I.

TABLE I. CAUCASIAN AND BANTU ATHLETES COMPARED WITH FIT YOUNG MEN

	Age (years)	Height (cm.)	Weight (kg.)
Caucasian athletes			
1. Richard C.	18	172·1	68·3
2. John V.	20	176·5	72·3
3. Wilhelm O.	28	179·0	62·3
4. Perry L.	24	184·1	67·3
Mean	23	177·9	67·5
Bantu athletes			
5. Daniel M.	33	—	50·5
6. John Q.	24	167·5	58·9
7. Benoni M.	23	177·7	69·6
8. Bennet M.	29	166·8	55·0
9. Humphrey K.	26	163·2	61·4
10. Thomas K.	23	163·2	55·2
Mean	25	167·7	58·4
Fit, young men			
Caucasian (N = 35)	19	175·9	71·8
Bantu (N = 88)	Young adults (No registration of births)	165·9	59·1

RESULTS

Pulmonary Ventilation

The pulmonary ventilations in l./min. (BTPS) of some 35 Caucasians and 88 Bantu who carried out the step test at four rates, were plotted against oxygen consumptions. Separate regression lines were fitted to the data for the Caucasians and the Bantu and these lines are shown in Fig. 1. The 83% confidence limits are relatively wide, compared with those fitted to

TABLE II. BANTU AND CAUCASIAN ATHLETES COMPARED

Subjects	Max. HR (beats/min.)	Pulm. vent. l./min.	BTPS	Max. oxygen l./min.	ml./kg./min.	Performance
1. Richard C.	192	—	140·8	4·07	59·6	Fastest 500 yard swim at 6,000 ft. altitude.
2. John V.	192	—	163·2	4·31	59·6	¼ mile—1 min. 53 sec.
3. Wilhelm O.	168	—	143·3	3·97	63·7	1 mile—4 min. 8 sec. / 2 miles—8 min. 53 sec. / 3 miles—13 min. 38 sec.
4. Perry L.	190	—	152·3	4·16	61·9	1 mile—4 min. 11 sec. / 3 miles—14 min. 28 sec.
Mean	186					
5. Daniel M.	190	—	149·9	4·13	61·2	3 miles—14 min. 11 sec.
		—	141·6	3·40	67·3	6 miles—29 min. 23 sec.
6. John Q.	192	—	151·4	3·84	65·2	¼ mile—1 min. 52 sec. / 1 mile—4 min. 12 sec.
7. Benoni M.	192	—	160·5	3·90	60·4	¼ mile—1 min. 48·7 sec.
8. Bennet M.	204	—	142·6	3·37	61·3	2 miles—9 min. 14·8 sec. / 3 miles—14 min. 14·7 sec.
9. Humphrey K.	204	—	163·8	3·46	56·4	½ mile—1 min. 48·7 sec.
10. Thomas K.	204	—	135·9	3·80	68·7	2 miles—9 min. 20 sec. / 3 miles—14 min. 19·8 sec.
Mean	198		149·5	3·69	63·2	

the regression lines of oxygen consumption against work rate, and overlap throughout, so that it can be concluded that the pulmonary ventilations of Caucasians and Bantu during physical effort at an altitude of 6,000 feet are not significantly different. The 'ventilatory equivalent'—the pulmonary ventilation (BTPS)/litre per min. of oxygen consumption—is approximately 30 litres.

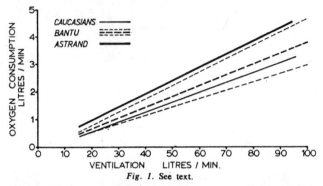

Fig. 1. See text.

Astrand's[2] regression line for ventilation against oxygen consumption at sea-level is also shown in Fig. 1. The ventilatory equivalent from this regression line is about 20 l./min. It can be concluded therefore that the ventilatory equivalent at 6,000 ft. altitude is about 50% greater than it is at sea-level.

Maximum Oxygen Intake

Caucasian athletes were significantly taller than the Bantu, with mean heights of 177·9 cm. and 167·7 cm., respectively (Table I). The Caucasians were also significantly heavier, with a mean weight of 67·5 kg. compared with the 58·5 kg. of the Bantu (Table I).

The mean maximum oxygen intake of the Caucasians was 4·13 l./min. and this is significantly greater than the mean of the Bantu athletes, 3·69 l./min. However, when these figures are expressed per kg. of body-weight—the correct basis for comparing samples of different weight—the mean maximum oxygen intakes of Caucasians and Bantu athletes are similar, being 61·1 and 63·2 ml./kg./min. respectively (Table II).

The mean ventilations (BTPS) of the 2 groups at their respective maximal levels of exercise are not significantly different.

DISCUSSION

In Fig. 1, it is shown that pulmonary ventilation was markedly increased during physical effort in Johannesburg. From this figure it can be estimated that a man running at a maximum oxygen intake of 4·0 l./min. at sea-level will have a pulmonary ventilation of 100 l./min. When he runs in Johannesburg the same pulmonary ventilation will give him an oxygen consumption of only 3·0 l./min. This level of oxygen intake would certainly not be sufficient for him to run his race at the same pace as at sea-level. If he is to increase his pulmonary ventilation in Johannesburg to give an oxygen consumption of 4·0 l./min. (which might be essential to achieve the same time for the event as at sea-level) then he would require a pulmonary ventilation of 130 l./min. The higher level of pulmonary ventilation might cause pulmonary distress and force the man to reduce his speed.

It could be argued that the air is less dense at the altitude of Johannesburg and that this would allow the man to increase his pulmonary ventilation without the distress that the same increase would occasion at sea-level. This hypothesis, however, needs to be tested by experimentation.

There is indirect evidence that the increased pulmonary ventilation at medium altitude decreases the *maximum* oxygen intake. In Johannesburg the mean maximum oxygen intake of the athletes was found to be 62·2 ml./kg./min. (mean pulmonary ventilation 149·4 l./min.) compared with the sea-level value of Astrand's athletes,[3] a mean maximum oxygen intake of 72·8 ml./kg./min. (with a mean pulmonary ventilation of 119·8 l./min).

From this evidence it may be concluded that performances at the altitude of Mexico City would be markedly affected, but that there is little possibility of danger to life.

This paper is published with the permission of the Transvaal and Orange Free State Chamber of Mines, Johannesburg.

REFERENCES
1. Abrahams, Sir A. (1950): *Encyclopaedia of Medical Practice,* 2nd ed., pp. 302 - 309. London: Butterworth.
2. Astrand. P. O. (1952): *Experimental Studies of Physical Working Capacity in Relation to Sex and Age.* Copenhagen: Munksgaard.
3. *Idem* (1955): Nature (Lond.), **176**, 922.
4. Leary, P. W. and Wyndham, C. H. (1965): S. Afr. Med. J.. **39**. 651.
5. Maritz, J. S.. Morrison, J. F., Strydom, N. B., and Wyndham, C. H. (1961): Ergonomics, **4**, 97.
6. Wyndham, C. H. and Leary, W. P. (1966): S. Afr. Med. J., **40**, 984.
7. Wyndham, C. H., Strydom, N. B., Morrison, J. F. and Maritz, J. S. (1959): J. Appl. Physiol., **14**, 927.

Altitude and Skiing*
MERRITT H. STILES, M.D.

INTRODUCTION

Though skiing, except for low altitude touring, is characteristically a mountain activity, altitude is rarely a problem. The physiological principles involved are simple, though a detailed explanation may seem somewhat complex.

ALTITUDE ACCLIMATIZATION

Fundamentally, physical activity is dependent upon the utilization of atmospheric oxygen by muscle cells in the production of energy. As Knuttgen[1] has pointed out, this process involves a number of steps (Table I). Yet these steps, as involved and complex as they may seem, are concerned with oxygen transport, and hence are only preliminary to the subsequent phases of oxidative metabolism, with storage and usage of oxidative energy in the more comprehensive process of aerobic energy release.

From the standpoint of physical activity at altitude, the important factor is that the barometric pressure and the partial pressure of oxygen are lower than at sea level. At 7500 feet elevation, for example, higher than Eastern and Central skiing, though somewhat lower than the major Colorado areas, the partial pressure of oxygen is about 20 percent lower than at sea level. This is of no consequence in ordinary physical activity, which uses only a minor portion of an individual's oxygen capacity. Usual

*Presented February 3, 1971, Conference on Skiing Injuries, American Academy of Orthopedic Surgeons, Snowmass-at-Aspen, Colorado.

Blood Oxygen Saturation at sea level is 97% – at 7500 feet it is 94.7% – a decrease which is about equivalent to that of an individual at sea level who smokes more than ½ pack of cigarettes per day. Nor is it of consequence even in maximum effort which does not last over one and three-quarters to two minutes, as was demonstrated so well in the 800 metre running events at Mexico City in 1968. This is because oxygen debt, or anaerobic capacity, is the principal factor in short duration effort. Energy for muscular activity comes from the splitting of high energy compounds, adenosine triphosphate and creatine phosphate. Oxygen is essential to resynthesize these compounds; the oxygen deficit required for resynthesis is termed the alactic oxygen debt. When a high work load is continued over a longer period of time an added mechanism comes into play, the breakdown of glycogen with the release of energy and the formation of lactic acid, constituting the so-called lactacid oxygen debt. Various estimates of the total oxygen debt capacity have been made. The theory of its measurement is simple, but actual application presents difficulties and quite widely varying results have been reported. Dill and Saktor's value of 5 to 6 litres in well-conditioned athletes, approximate-

TABLE 1

DELIVERY OF ATMOSPHERIC OXYGEN TO MUSCLE CELLS
1. Delivery of air to alveoli by pulmonary ventilation
2. Diffusion of oxygen from alveoli to plasma through pulmonary membrane and capillary wall
3. Diffusion through red cell membrane and union with hemoglobin
4. Delivery to systemic capillaries through blood flow
5. Diffusion through red cell membrane to plasma
6. Delivery to tissue cells by diffusion and extracellular fluid flow
7. Diffusion through muscle cell membrane

ly equal to the maximum oxygen uptake for a period of a minute, is perhaps the most realistic estimate available.[2]

Even though it may be of little importance to the average skier, altitude acclimatization does occur, though the factors involved are not entirely understood. There is evidence to suggest that altitude acclimatization and conditioning at any altitude are only different phases of the same general process. Both produce a relative hypoxemia, followed by a series of adaptive changes.[3] Increased pulmonary ventilation, the most prompt in onset, has been most studied and written about. It long has been known that a decrease in the partial pressure of oxygen in the inspired air leads to an increase in ventilation through its effect on carotid and aortic chemoreceptors. There is no agreement, however, as to the altitude where this mechanism comes into play. While it has been stated that adaptive changes may occur at elevations as low as 1000 meters, most authorities place the critical altitude much higher. Van Liere and Stickney[4] state that in experienced subjects at rest there was no effect on the respiratory rate up to 10,000 feet, and only very minor increases up to 16,000 feet, with about 20 percent increase at 20,000 feet, but that with exercise there was a definite increase at 14,000 feet.

Yet it is generally agreed that there is considerable individual variation, and that many, if not most, lowlanders newly arrived at moderate altitude demonstrate increased ventilation which disappears with continued residence. This hyperventilation cannot be accounted for by any known chemical changes in the blood, and the probable role of neurogenic factors has been suggested by many authorities. As at sea level, hyperventilation leads to an alkalosis, which accounts for the symptoms experienced by many altitude newcomers. The hyperventilation, if persistent, may lead to transient phasic breathing,[5] particularly at night and even at moderate altitude. The cycles, which are shorter than is the rule in subjects with heart disease, are clearly related to hyperventilation, since hypocapnia is present even during the apneic phase.[5] It is of interest that inappropriate hyperventilation may even be present following strenuous exercise.[6]

With prolonged residence at altitude, the red blood cell mass is increased, and at elevations about 10,000 feet pulmonary hypertension develops.[7] In considering these changes, along with the increased ventilation, Hecht has stated: From the standpoint of the altitude dweller, sea level man is a pulmonary hypotensive, anemic hypoventilator.[5]

While there have been conflicting reports on the effect of altitude on cardiac output, there is agreement that the maximum oxygen uptake is decreased, because of the lower partial pressure of oxygen. There is agreement, further, that the oxygen uptake improves with training, most of the improvement coming within 10 to 14 days at moderate altitude. Increased hemoglobin and myoglobin, increased tissue vascularization and widened arteriovenous oxygen difference are factors in this improvement. There is evidence also that the anaerobic capacity may increase.[3]

CROSS COUNTRY SKI COMPETITION

Altitude has never been considered a problem in Alpine ski competition; competitive events are of short duration, and the effort required mostly submaximal. Altitude has been considered important, however, in cross country skiing, with an International Ski Federation regulation that cross country competition should not be held at altitudes higher than 1500 meters. It is true, of course, that any given cross country race would require a longer running time at an altitude above 1500 meters than it would at a lower altitude, just as would any prolonged event requiring maximal effort. Studies related to the XIX Olympiad demonstrated clearly that, while performance times may be prolonged in competition at higher altitudes, all contestants are equally affected, there is no danger which does not exist at lower altitudes, and altitude acclimatization in a well-conditioned athlete does not require more than two to three weeks. While it is my feeling that the archaic FIS restriction on cross country competition should be discarded, my recommendation to this effect, at the International Colloquy on Medical Problems Related to Championship Skiing,[8] held at Grenoble in 1968, has had no noticeable effect.

PULMONARY EDEMA OF ALTITUDE

Our discussion up to this point has suggested that any altitude discomfort experienced by the average Alpine skier is psychological rather than physiological. As an aside, some of you may have had difficulty in selling this idea to acquaintances, as I have. I recall particularly two persons, one a Professor of Cardiology at a prestigious Eastern school who refused to believe that the symptoms he had experienced riding in a car at 7500 feet elevation might have been the result of subconscious hyperventilation, the other an intelligent professional who refused to admit that the discomforting symptoms she always experienced during her first two to three days at Vail were psychological in origin, until she remembered that she never had any trouble at Aspen.

There are occasional physiological problems which may affect the high altitude skier, the most serious being pulmonary edema. This is a rare, and still rather mysterious, disorder which occurs in the unacclimatized sea level dweller who ascends rapidly to an elevation above 10,000 feet and engages in heavy, often unaccustomed, physical activity as mountain climbing, armed combat, and, very rarely, skiing. Strangely, it is more frequent in previously acclimatized altitude dwellers who return to altitude after a sojourn of ten days or more at sea level.[9]

157

The first symptoms, which appear from 6 to 36 hours after arrival at altitude, consist of a dry cough, dyspnea, weakness, and pain or pressure in the lower substernal area.[10] Anorexia, nausea and vomiting, may appear. Later respiration becomes noisy with audible wheezing; bubbling rales are present. Orthopnea and hemoptysis may develop. In severe cases, chest x-ray reveals confluent or nodular densities, bilateral or unilateral. Central pulmonary vessels are full and the pulmonary arteries may be prominent. The electrocardiogram may show changes suggestive of right ventricular strain.

While some features suggest pneumonia, there is little if any leucocytosis, the sedimentation rate is normal and antibiotics are ineffective. On the other hand, bed rest and oxygen therapy, best under positive pressure, or return to lower altitude, bring prompt relief.

Cardiac catheterization during the acute stage has revealed marked pulmonary hypertension, a low cardiac output, and normal pulmonary wedge pressure. The calculated pulmonary arteriolar resistance is markedly elevated, compatible with arteriolar constriction. Oxygen therapy results in a prompt fall in pulmonary artery pressure.

The mechanism of edema formation is not known. The elevated pulmonary artery pressure may be a factor, yet it is a normal occurrence found in all persons at higher altitudes. Blount and Vogel found the pulmonary artery pressure normal at 7500 feet in normal subjects, but elevated at 10,000 feet, 25 mm in comparison with 15 mm at Denver's 5000 feet. The difference was still greater with exercise, 12 − 16 mm at 5000, and 25 − 54 mm at 10,000 feet. The rise in pulmonary artery pressure was gradual going from 5000 to 10,000 feet, but more rapid in going from 5000 to 14,000 feet.[7]

Pulmonary edema of altitude is readily distinguished from acute mountain sickness, which comes on immediately on arrival at altitude rather than after a delay of 6 or more hours. Yet it has been speculated that the hyperventilation of the altitude newcomer coupled with severe exercise hyperventilation might deplete lung surfactants, which, combined with exertional distention of the capillary bed, might favor alveolar fluid escape in susceptible persons.[11]

Regardless of the pathogenetic mechanism, acute pulmonary edema is rare. Yet its remote risk for the average skier still emphasizes the importance of adequate physical conditioning prior to a skiing expedition at high altitude, and it suggests that the poorly-conditioned lowlander who is planning a high altitude ski vacation might be well advised to spend a day or two skiing at moderate altitude enroute to his high altitude destination. It has been suggested that a couple of days rest at high altitude might be helpful before engaging in active exercise. This recommendation leaves me unenthusiastic, in view of the rapid deterioration which follows even short periods of inactivity.[12]

ACUTE MOUNTAIN SICKNESS

Newcomers to altitude may exhibit a variety of symptoms: headache, insomnia, malaise, unrest, lassitude, apathy or heightened irritability, incoordination, diminution of visual acuity, decrease in auditory perception, muscular weakness, fatigability, disturbances in breathing, tachycardia and lack of appetite. These symptoms, which begin to appear immediately on arrival at altitude, are grouped under the term "acute mountain sickness." They are assumed to be primarily the result of subconscious hyperventilation and alkalosis. The skier who experiences such symptoms might just as well laugh them off and go on his way; there is no specific cure, though possibly rebreathing to avoid the loss of even more carbon dioxide might be of benefit.

CHRONIC MOUNTAIN SICKNESS

Chronic Mountain Sickness, also called Seroché or Mongé's Disease, is another story. It is found only after prolonged residence at higher elevations; it is characterized by excessive erythrocytosis, beyond the expected altitude response. The symptoms in some respects are similar to those encountered in polycythemia and in syndromes associated with alveolar hypoventilation at sea level, notably severe obesity, constrictive airway disease, or post-encephalitic syndrome. The few studies available suggest the syndrome may be an example of alveolar hypoventilation at altitude, initiated by an apparent loss of chemoreceptor drives resulting in relative hypoventilation, hypercapnia and erythrocytosis.[13] Symptoms are relieved promptly by descent to a lower altitude.

Chronic mountain sickness should not be a problem to the Alpine skier unless he chooses to reverse the usual skier pattern, skiing at customary altitudes but then ascending a mountain to spend the rest of his time at much higher elevations.

REFERENCES

1. Knuttgen, H. G.: Physical Working Capacity and Physical Performance, Med. and Sci. in Sports, 1: 1-8 (March) 1969.
2. Dill, D. B. and Saktor, B.: Exercise and the Oxygen Debt, J. Sports Med., 2: 66-72 (June) 1962.
3. Stiles, M. H.: Training for Competition at Moderate Altitude, Conference on Hypoxia, High Altitude and the Heart, Aspen Adv. Cardiology, Vol. 5,   , Karger, New York.
4. VanLiere, E. J. and Stickney, J. C.: Hypoxia, p 126, (University Chicago Press 1963).
5. Hecht, H. H.: Certain Vascular Adjustments and Maladjustments at Altitudes. Exercise and Altitude, p 134-148, Jokl and Jokl (eds), S. Bargen, 1968.
6. Ferguson, A., Addington, W. W. and Guensler, E. A.: Dyspnea and Bronchospasm from Inappropriate Postexercise Hyperventilation, Ann. Int. Med. 71, p 1063-1072, (Dec.) 1969.
7. Blount, S. G. Jr. and Vogel, J. H. K.: Altitude and Pulmonary Hypertension, Exercise and Altitude, p 149-154, Jokl and Jokl (eds), S. Barger, 1968.
8. Stiles, M. H.: Training and Competition at Moderate Altitudes, Proceedings 2nd International Colloquy on Medical Problems Connected with Championship Skiing, p 39-41, Grenoble, 1968.
9. Penaloza, D. and Sims, F.: Circulatory Dynamics during High Altitude Pulmonary Edema, Am. Jr. Cardiology 23, 369-378 (March) 1969.
10. Hultgren, H. N.: High Altitude Pulmonary Edema, Proceedings of International Symposium of the Effects of Altitude on Physical Performance, p 53-56. R. F. Goddard, ed., The Athletic Institute, Chicago, 1967.
11. Singh, I., Kapila, C. C., Khauna, P. K., Nanda, R. B. and Rao, B. B. B.: Pulmonary Edema, Exercise and Altitude, p 165-179, Jokl and Jokl (eds.) S. Barger, 1968.
12. Saltin, B., Blomquist, G., Mitchell, J. H., Johnson, R. L. Jr., Wildenthal, K. and Chapman, C. B.: Response to Exercise after Bed Rest and after Training, Circulation 38, Supp. 7. p 1-78 (Nov.) 1968.
13. Mongé, C., Locano, R. and Carcelon, A.: Renal Excretion of Bicarbonate, Jr. Clin. Invest. 43, p 2303-2309 (Dec.) 1964.

Effect of Exercise on Thyroxine Degradation in Athletes and Non-athletes

C. H. G. IRVINE

A NUMBER of writers have investigated (1–8) or discussed (9, 10) the quantitative relationship between thyroid activity and muscular activity. While Bondy and Hagewood (2) found that in rats two hours' swimming caused a pronounced fall in protein-bound iodine, in a later report from the same laboratory Lashof et al. (3) commented that the low "temperature of the water rather than the muscular activity may have been enough to account for the fall in PBI." Escobar del Rey and Morreale de Escobar (7) found that, three hours after thyroxine ^{131}I, resting rats had a significantly lower plasma PB^{131}I than those which swam vigorously for most of the period. On the other hand, when slaughtered at the end of 24 hours, resting rats had a significantly higher plasma PB^{131}I than rats which ran for nine of the 24 hours (8). Most other evidence suggests that muscular activity has no relationship (3, 5, 6) or an inverse relationship (1, 4, 10) to thyroid activity. Recently, Gregerman et al. (9) concluded that "an unequivocal answer is not presently possible." In a group of horses Irvine (11) found that, after a three-month course of physical training, the thyroxine secretion rate had increased to 165%, and fractional turnover had increased to 265% of pretraining values. In this report quantitative relationship between muscular activity and thyroxine degradation is compared in athletes and non-athletes.

Materials and Methods

Subjects were healthy young men between the ages of 18 and 25 and were divided into 3 groups. The first group consisted of 10 track athletes who had just completed their track season but had agreed to continue training at a moderate intensity for a further 2 weeks. Training consisted of a 30–45 min exercise period with energy output at 640 kcal. This is about half the energy expenditure of these athletes when in intensive training just prior to the commencement of this experiment. This experiment continued for 5 days. In 3 athletes observations were continued for a further 3 days during which no exercise was taken. The second group consisted of 6 controls who had not recently engaged in any physical exertion. The third group of 12 had not engaged in any athletics or other exertion more strenuous than billiards for some months prior to the experiment, and for the last month had avoided all but minimal physical activity. On the sixth day of the experiment, this group was subdivided into 2 equal groups. Subgroup a served as controls while subgroup b undertook each day a $\frac{3}{4}$ hr period of exercise, at the end of which they had reached a fatigue level comparable with that of the exercising athletes. This experiment concluded after a further 6 days. All groups undertook little activity outside the exercise period. Temperatures were in the range 10–21 C throughout. All subjects were given daily 1–4 mg potassium iodide for 1 week prior to the experiment in an attempt to reduce the specific activity of endogenous thyroxine ^{131}I without affecting peripheral

TABLE 1. Thyroxine metabolism in trained athletes and untrained controls

No.	Weight kg	PBI μg/100 ml	TDS liters	T₄ pool mg I⁻	k	TSR/day μg I⁻	Free T₄%
a. Athletes							
1	65.8	6.0	11.58	0.695	.190	132	0.066
2	57.7	5.2	11.50	0.598	0.168	100	0.046
5	61.7	4.8	10.91	0.525	0.165	87	0.040
6	67.1	6.0	11.63	0.698	0.154	108	0.050
7	69.4	5.6	11.77	0.660	0.169	111	0.051
8	59.0	6.5	11.00	0.715	0.149	107	0.044
9	62.2	6.1	11.63	0.710	0.159	113	0.046
10	64.5	5.5	11.77	0.648	0.171	111	0.060
11	68.6	4.8	12.07	0.580	0.183	106	0.052
12	57.7	6.2	11.00	0.682	0.175	119	0.040
Mean	63.37	5.67	11.49	0.652	0.168	109	0.050
SD	4.376	0.592	0.387	0.0677	0.0125	11.7	0.0085
b. Controls							
1	69.8	5.8	11.23	0.653	0.089	58	0.037
2	68.0	5.2	11.12	0.579	0.103	60	0.046
3	65.8	6.0	11.00	0.660	0.099	66	0.040
4	63.5	6.2	10.87	0.675	0.114	77	0.051
5	61.2	6.1	10.64	0.661	0.104	69	0.043
6	59.8	5.0	10.42	0.521	0.093	48	0.037
Mean	64.68	5.72	10.88	0.623	0.100	62	0.042
SD	3.894	0.50	0.0346	0.00612	0.0088	10	0.0057

thyroxine metabolism.

Five to 20 μc of thyroxine [131]I (Radiochemical Centre, England) was given into the right median cubital vein and blood was collected from the corresponding left vein every 24 hr and occasionally more frequently, as indicated later. Ninety-four per cent of the dose of ^{131}I was found by paper chromatography to be in the form of thyroxine. In athletes thyroxine turnover curves were based on pre-exercise samples. In athletes, zinc hydroxide precipitable ^{131}I, and in all other subjects total serum ^{131}I, was counted on 3 ml aliquots in a spectrometer to an accuracy of $\pm 2\%$. This ^{131}I was found by paper chromatography of concentrated butanol extracts of plasma to be over 95% thyroxine. Percentage of the administered dose in 1 liter of plasma was calculated by comparison with an aliquot of the dose injected and plotted against time. Zero time concentration was obtained by extrapolation of the smooth exponential curve obtained from at least 4 points during the 2–5 day period. This necessitated extra collection in subjects whose 48 hr count indicated that the thyroxine ^{131}I had not equilibrated. Daily fractional over of pool (FT) was obtained using the same values. Protein-bound iodine (PBI) was estimated as described elsewhere (12) and the extrathyroidal thyroxine iodine pool calculated as the product of the distribution space in liters (TDS) (reciprocal of zero-time concentration) and PBI/liter. The amount of thyroxine iodine degraded/day is the product of the fractional turnover and the thyroxine pool. As PBI was not significantly changed in any subject during the experimental period, degradation rate may also be regarded as the isotope dilution rate or thyroxine secretion rate (TSR). Percentage free thyroxine was measured by the method of Sterling and Brenner (13). In the athletes the percentage free thyroxine and PBI were estimated on samples taken while they were in full training, 1 week prior to isotope administration and just prior to the commencement of iodide administration. In groups 2 and 3 PBI was measured both 1 week prior to and at the end of the experiment. Total urine collections were made and ^{131}I counted in both exercised and non-exercised subjects of the third group on the 11th and 12th days after isotope administration. Organic and inorganic urinary ^{131}I were sepa-

164

rated by an ion-exchange resin, the separation efficiency of which was determined by adding thyroxine ^{125}I or iodide ^{125}I to the urine.

Results

In most subjects who exercised up to four hours after isotope administration, the 24-hour plasma thyroxine ^{131}I fell on or slightly below the curve extrapolated from later measurements. In resting subjects, on the other hand, the 24-hour value was up to 15% above the curve, while the 48-hour value was occasionally elevated. This is taken to indicate that, as a result of exercise, equilibration of thyroxine ^{131}I in the thyroxine space is accelerated, and is completed before 24 hours. Five daily measurements on a straight line were thus available in athletes (Fig. 1).

Thyroxine degradation/secretion rates are given in Table 1 and thyroxine fractional turnover rates in Table 2. Thyroxine degradation/secretion rate is 75% higher and thyroxine fractional turnover is 68% higher when physically trained subjects engaging in moderately strenuous exercise are compared with untrained subjects not engaging in exercise. Application of Student's t-test shows this change in both measurements to be highly significant (p <0.001). PBI did not differ significantly. Thyroxine distribution space was 5.6% higher in athletes (p <0.01). The 19% higher free thyroxine percentage and the 17% higher absolute free thyroxine in the athletes were not statistically significant (p <0.10 >0.05). A group of three of these athletes ceased training for three days. Mean fractional turnover had fallen from 0.171 to 0.133 by the third day. However, as the latter figure is determined from three samples 12 hours apart, it should be regarded as only a qualitative rather than a quanti-

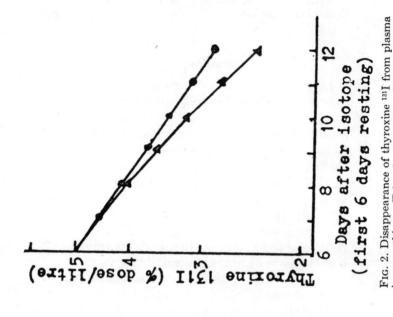

Fig. 2. Disappearance of thyroxine ^{131}I from plasma in non-athletes. Triangle = exercising daily (n = 6); circle = resting (n = 6).

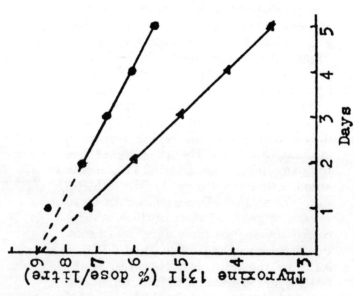

Fig. 1. Disappearance of thyroxine ^{131}I from plasma. Triangle = athlete exercising daily; circle = non-athlete resting.

tative indication of the effect of cessation of activity.

In the third group, mean fractional turnover of 0.097 during the resting period is slightly lower than that of the second group and 10% lower than the figure calculated for the same age and sex from the data of Oddie et al. (14). The nature of their data does not permit statistical comparison with the present results. Over the period of these experiments (12 days), the disappearance of thyroxine ^{131}I from plasma is usually represented as a simple exponential. In these experiments the slope became slightly more horizontal with time but the difference between the first and second six-day periods was not significant. However, in the exercised subgroup turnover increased steadily over the second six-day period, being 7% greater over the first two days (NS), 28% greater over the second two days (p < 0.05), and 44% greater over the final two days (p < 0.01). While the turnover measurements over these two-day periods may lack precision, being dependent on only three samples which did not fall on a straight line, over the whole six-day period during which six samples were taken, turnover rate is 33% higher than in resting controls (Fig. 2).

Data obtained from urinary collection in non-athletes show that, in the exercising group, urinary ^{131}I excretion over the fifth and sixth days of exercise was 34% greater than over the same period in resting controls (p < 0.01) (Table 3). In both groups, approximately 94% of the ^{131}I was inorganic.

Discussion

Lewallen et al. (15) have discussed errors in multiple pool turnover studies using tracers, as in the present method. As ap-

TABLE 2. Thyroxine fractional turnover in athletes and non-athletes

	No. of subjects	Fractional turnover	SD
Athletes			
In training	3*	0.171	0.0120
After 3 days' rest	3*	0.133	0.121–0.142†
Non-athletes			
Resting, unselected	6	0.100	0.0088
Resting, selected			
Subgroup a			
During days 0–6	6	0.097	0.0071
During days 6–12	6	0.094	0.0069
Subgroup b			
During days 0–6	6	0.097	0.0112
Exercising, selected			
Subgroup b			
During days 6–8 (first 2 days' exer.)	6	0.105	0.0095
During days 8–10 (second 2 days' exer.)	6	0.125	0.0075
During days 10–12 (third 2 days' exer.)	6	0.140	0.0090
During days 6–12	6	0.125	

* Identical subjects.
† Range.

plied to the present study these would result in: (a) Incorrect estimation of the thyroxine distribution space and consequently TSR. This arises from inequality in rates of isotope secretion from compartments with different exchange rates when the early, equilibrating phase and the late, post-equilibration phase are compared. (b) The assumption that the fractional turnover of the whole pool is equal to the fractional turnover of plasma. As will be shown elsewhere, these are sources of error in the present paper resulting in overestimation of the TSR by approximately 15% in resting non-athletes, according to the equations of Lewallen *et al.* However, because major difficulties are introduced when these equations are applied to a system disturbed by muscular exercise early in the equilibration phase, it has been decided to use the method described. This permits comparison of data obtained under varied conditions of these experiments as the error is relatively constant throughout. The complex problem of kinetic analysis during a disturbed equilibration phase will be discussed elsewhere.

From Tables 1 and 2, it is concluded that muscular exercise causes an increase in thyroxine secretion and degradation rate resulting from increased fractional turnover with little change in pool size. This may arise primarily from central causes which result in increased secretion by the gland, or from peripheral causes which result in increased degradation. Central causes should result in an increase in the absolute free thyroxine level. Although a mean increase of 17% was found in these experiments, it was not significant. De Nayer *et al.* (16) have found a normal free thyroxine level in athletes in training. Therefore, it seems likely that the major part of the increase is primarily due to increased pe-

169

ripheral degradation. It would be more appropriate to describe the change as increased thyroxine degradation rather than secretion. The increase in urinary ^{131}I iodide indicates that the increased degradation is largely if not wholly due to increased deiodination rather than degradation via some other route in which iodide is not an end-product.

The results suggest that athletes have a faster thyroxine turnover than non-athletes undertaking the same exercise and at the end of a three-day rest period have a faster turnover than resting non-athletes. It may be considered that subjects capable of highly successful athletic endeavor, as these were, may have an inherently higher rate of thyroxine metabolism. In experiments of this type, it is desirable that each subject serve as his own control to assess this possibility. Unfortunately, these athletes could not be measured in the untrained state as they trained to some extent all the year round. However, from the marked increase in turnover in unselected non-athletes who commenced taking exercise, and from the decrease in turnover when athletes ceased taking exercise, the conclusion that exercise *per se* does increase thyroxine turnover and degradation rate seems justified. The increase in thyroxine distribution space may be related to the increase of 20 to 40% in plasma volume commonly observed in trained athletes (17). The third group had a low thyroxine fractional turnover compared with the figures calculated for comparable randomly selected subjects in the report of Oddie *et al.* (14). However, when volunteers for this group were being requested, it was emphasized that only physically inactive subjects were required for this group. It cannot therefore be claimed that subjects were randomly selected in respect to physical

TABLE 3. Urinary excretion of ^{131}I after thyroxine ^{131}I in exercising and resting non-athletes

	5th and 6th day of exercise (11th and 12th days after isotope)	Resting (11th and 12th days after isotope)
No. of subjects	5	6
Plasma ^{131}I levels at 48 hr intervals (% dose/liter)	2.96 – 2.24	3.23 – 2.67
Fall in plasma ^{131}I (% dose/liter)	0.72	0.56
TDS (liters)	11.92	11.70
Loss from TDS over 48 hr as % dose given	8.64	6.54
Urinary recovery over 48 hr as % dose given	6.06	4.96
Daily excretion of hormonally derived iodine (µg)	66 ±10.6*	49 ±7.9*

* SD.

activity in that, mostly by choice, they had been taking no part in physical activities common to young male adults, and also undertook minimum activity before and during the experiment. While Reichlin *et al.* (4) have found that inactivity caused by drugs or physical disease did not lower thyroxine turnover, no reference could be found to the effects of physical inertia on thyroxine metabolism in healthy subjects.

While the results of these experiments appear to be at variance with the conclusions of previous workers, this may be due to difference in approach. The relationship between thyroid function and muscular exercise has been assessed previously by (a) difference between pre- and post-exercise PBI in intact (2, 3, 5) and thyroid-ectomized, thyroxine-replaced (2, 7, 8) subjects, (b) labeled thyroxine turnover rate (3, 4), (c) thyroidal ^{131}I uptake, $PB^{131}I$ and RBC uptake of triiodothyronine (1, 6).

Interpretation of these tests is subject to many variables. These include:

a. The inconsistency with which water movements during and immediately after exercise cause an increased concentration in plasma protein-bound substances with no real movements of the substance itself. This increase, which in strenuous exercise may reach 15% (5, 6), usually peaks at $\frac{1}{2}$ hour, with return to normal by $1\frac{1}{2}$ hours.

b. The varying response time of the feedback mechanism, and possible overshoot.

c. Diffusion of albumin into extravascular spaces during exercise and its slow return by lymphatics is known to occur during severe exercise. If, as some believe (18), the smaller thyroxine-binding globulin molecule behaves similarly, temporary changes in the level of PBI unrelated to thyroxine metabolism would occur.

d. The acute psychic stress which accompanied exercise in some reports (1, 5) would, according to present concepts, result in sufficient depression of thyroid function to mask the effects of exercise *per se* (10).

e. In the horse a latent period in excess of ten days occurs between commencement of regular physical exercise and the development of a marked increase in thyroxine turnover (11). The present experiments indicate a shorter latent period in man.

f. The intensity, duration and frequency of the exercise are important. Workers measuring labeled thyroxine turnover have confined their observations to either (i) the difference between ambulatory subjects and those in whom immobility resulted either from physical disease or prolonged sleep induced by drugs (4), or (ii) the difference between turnover on a day during which subjects walked for four hours, and the average daily turnover when this exercise was not taken. From Table 2 it may be seen that the change in slope of the plasma disappearance curve after one day's vigorous exercise was below minimum response (20%) claimed for the method in this report (3).

The failure of these workers to obtain an effect due to muscular exercise is not surprising in view of the inadequacy of the exercise or the insensitivity of the method.

Wilson's subjects undertook strenuous manual labor for five weeks, after which he concluded that "measurements gave no evidence of pituitary or thyroid stimulation as an after effect of continued exposure to increased physical activity." He based this on absence of any change in PBI, RBC uptake of triiodothyronine, or per cent uptake of ^{131}I by the thyroid. However, he observed a 40 to 50% increase in food intake without any change in the nature of the diet, which suggests that absolute iodine uptake was increased by 40 to 50%. As the thyroidal iodine pool decreased during the training period, this is consistent with a greatly accelerated iodine loss from the thyroid. Wilson gave ^{131}I iodide to his subjects both before and after training, measuring PB^{131}I after 4, 24 and 48 hours. It is interesting to note that in the trained subject, the PB^{131}I reached much higher levels than in the untrained. At four hours it was ten times higher and although PB^{131}I fell steadily after this, it was still four to five times higher in the trained than untrained subjects at 48 hours. This fall from four hours onward, compared with a steady increase in controls, suggests rapid iodine turnover, both in the gland and peripherally as hormone. Under the circumstances, his failure to find an altered thyroidal uptake could be consistent with a very brief stay in the gland, rather than unaltered thyroidal iodine metabolism. This, in conjunction with increased iodine intake, might well be interpreted as showing that thyroid function is increased in manual labor.

References

1. Bogoroch, R., and P. Timiras, *Endocrinology* **49**: 548, 1951.
2. Bondy, P. K., and M. A. Hagewood, *Proc Soc Exp Biol Med* **81**: 328, 1952.
3. Lashof, J. C., P. K. Bondy, K. Sterling, and E. B. Man, *Proc Soc Exp Biol Med* **86**: 233, 1954.
4. Reichlin, S., M. G. Koussa, and F. W. Witt, *J Clin Endocr* **19**: 692, 1959.
5. Volpe, R., J. Vale, and W. J. MacAllister, *J Clin Endocr* **20**: 415, 1960.
6. Wilson, O., *Fed Proc* **25**: 1357, 1966.
7. Escobar del Rey, F., and G. Morreale de Escobar, *Acta Endocr (Kobenhavn)* **23**: 393, 1956.
8. ————, *Ibid.*, p. 400.
9. Gregerman, R. J., G. W. Gaffney, and N. W. Shock, *J Clin Invest* **41**: 2065, 1962.
10. Donovan, B. T., *Brit Med Bull* **22**: 249, 1966.
11. Irvine, C. H. G., *J Endocr* **39**: 313, 1967.
12. ————, *Amer J Vet Res* **28**: 1687, 1967.

13. Sterling, K., and M. A. Brenner, *J Clin Invest* **45:** 153, 1966.
14. Oddie, T. H., J. H. Meade, Jr., and D. A. Fisher, *J Clin Endocr* **26:** 425, 1966.
15. Lewallen, C. G., M. Berman, and J. E. Rall, *J Clin Invest* **38:** 66, 1959.
16. De Nayer, P., P. Malvaux, M. Ostyn, H. G. Van den Schrieck, and M. De Visscher, *Trav Soc Med Belge Educ Phys Sports* **18:** 1, 1965.
17. Steinhaus, A. H., *Physiol Rev* **13:** 103, 1933.

METABOLIC FUELS DURING AND AFTER SEVERE EXERCISE IN ATHLETES AND NON-ATHLETES

R. H. JOHNSON   J. L. WALTON

H. A. KREBS   D. H. WILLIAMSON

Summary   Training of athletes has been shown to affect in a major way the metabolism of fat and carbohydrate during and after exercise. The concentrations of acetoacetate, 3-hydroxybutyrate, free fatty acids (F.F.A.), glycerol, lactate, pyruvate, and glucose were measured in the blood of nine athletes and eighteen non-athletes before, during, and after running for $1^1/_2$ hours. Measurements were also made of speed of running, weight loss, and heart-rate. There were striking differences in metabolite concentrations between the two groups. The concentrations of lactate and pyruvate did not rise in the group of athletes during the initial period of exercise. The untrained group developed post-exercise ketosis which was associated with high F.F.A. concentrations. The F.F.A. concentrations increased much less in the athletes during exercise, and consequently in the recovery period they had relatively low ketone-body concentrations. So, in general, the metabolite concentrations in the blood of athletes deviate less from normal during exercise than those of untrained subjects.

Introduction

THE cause of post-exercise ketosis, a form of ketosis first reported by Courtice and Douglas,[1] is not yet clearly understood. A new approach to the problem was suggested by the finding that post-exercise ketosis seemed to depend on the athletic training of the exercised subject. The majority of a group of hill walkers who were fit, but not in athletic training, gave a positive test for acetoacetate in the urine (' Ketostix ' method) after 3–5 hours of walking,[2] whereas runners after competing in a marathon race (42 km.) gave a negative test even though the exercise had been more strenuous [3]; likewise, Astrand et al.[4] found no ketonuria in competitors after an 85 km. ski race.

We have investigated the effect of training on post-exercise ketosis by measuring the concentration of metabolites (acetoacetate, 3-hydroxybutyrate, free fatty acids, glycerol, lactate, pyruvate, and glucose) in the blood of trained and untrained subjects before, during, and after exercise.

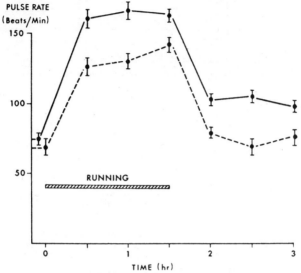

Fig. 1—Mean and S.E.M. of heart-rates of athletes (●········●) and untrained subjects (●————●) before, during, and after running for $1^1/_2$ hours.

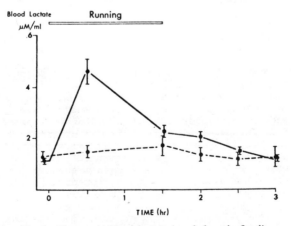

Fig. 2—Changes in blood-lactate (symbols as in fig. 1).

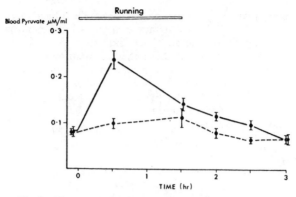

Fig. 3—Changes in blood-pyruvate (symbols as in fig. 1).

Methods

Subjects

Nine subjects (aged 22–34 years) trained regularly to compete in running events of between 15–42 km., by running 60–150 km. per week. Their mean ($\pm$ S.D.) weight was 64·3 ($\pm$ 3·5) kg., and height 174·5 ($\pm$ 6·1) cm. The eighteen untrained subjects (aged 20–23 years) were university students who did not participate regularly in any athletic sport and were not in training. Their mean weight was 68·1 ($\pm$ 8·0) kg., and mean height 176·0 ($\pm$ 8·3) cm.

Procedure

The investigations were done between 11 A.M. and 8 P.M., and all were started about 3 hours after the previous meal. They were carried out on mild, dry days with temperatures varying between 17 and 22°C, with little wind (calm to force 2), and light cloud cover.

The subjects ran for periods of $1^1/_2$ hours on an outdoor track; lap-times were recorded and observations were then continued for a further 2 hours. They were asked to choose their own running speed. They were weighed before and after exercise. Radial pulse-rates were measured before running, and at 30-minute intervals during and after exercise. During the period of exercise, the subjects stopped for about 4 minutes every 30 minutes and pulse-rates were recorded for the immediate 30 seconds after stopping running.

Blood-samples (15 ml.) were taken by venepuncture before running, 30 minutes later, at the end of exercise, and then at 30-minute intervals. In some cases, blood-samples were also taken at 30-minute intervals during the exercise period. Each blood-sample was divided into two parts; 5 ml. was immediately added to 5 ml. of 10% perchloric acid, and the remainder was added to a heparin tube, and the plasma separated by centrifugation. All samples were then stored in ice. After removal of protein and neutralisation with potassium hydroxide, the perchloric acid sample was analysed by enzymatic methods for acetoacetate and 3-hydroxybutyrate,[5] lactate and pyruvate,[6] glucose,[7] and glycerol.[8] The plasma sample was analysed for free fatty acids (F.F.A.).[9]

The results are expressed in the text as means and standard deviations.

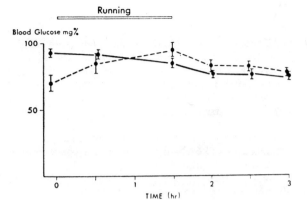

Fig. 4—Changes in blood-glucose (symbols as in fig. 1).

Results

The athletes ran much faster (16±2 km. per hour) than the untrained group (10±3 km. per hour), and they ran at a steady speed, whereas the others showed considerable variation and slowed down progressively. The athletes lost more weight (3·29±0·36% total body-weight) than the non-athletes (1·80±0·43% total body-weight). The mean heart-rates of the athletes were lower than those of the untrained subjects. After ½ hour and 1 hour of exercise, the athletes and non-athletes had mean heart-rates of 126 and 130, and 160 and 165 beats per minute, respectively. Half an

MEAN (± S.D.) CONCENTRATIONS OF METABOLITES IN ATHLETES
AND NON-ATHLETES AT REST AND AFTER RUNNING FOR 30 MINUTES

Metabolite*	Athletes		Non-athletes	
	At rest	After 30 min. exercise	At rest	After 30 min. exercise
Lactate ..	1·31±0·53	1·49±0·62	1·14±0·41	4·63±2·05
Pyruvate ..	0·079±0·029	0·099±0·035	0·081±0·023	0·234±0·087
Glucose ..	3·97±1·00	4·78±1·17	5·20±0·64	5·11±0·82
Glycerol ..	0·051±0·016	0·176±0·061	0·072±0·022	0·165±0·060
F.F.A. ..	0·36±0·13	0·45±0·19	0·53±0·33	0·65±0·39
Ketone bodies	0·062±0·009	0·089±0·032	0·081±0·025	0·125±0·045

* All in μmole per ml. except for plasma-F.F.A. which is expressed in μeq. per ml. 1 μmole glucose per ml. is equivalent to 18 mg. per 100 ml.

hour after exercise, the mean heart-rates were 78 and 102 beats per minute, respectively (fig. 1).

Concentrations of Metabolites in Blood during and after Exercise

Metabolite levels before, during, and after exercise are shown in figs. 2–7; mean (± S.D.) levels at rest and after 30 minutes of running are summarised in the table.

Lactate.—Resting blood-lactate levels were similar in both groups. During the exercise, the greatest difference between the two groups was in the early stages. After 30 minutes, the athletes had a mean level of 1·49 ($\pm$ 0·62) µmole per ml.; in the non-athletes the lactate concentrations had risen to 4·63 ($\pm$ 2·05) µmole per ml. after 30 minutes, decreasing thereafter throughout the rest of the experiment (fig. 2).

Pyruvate.—The changes in pyruvate concentration were similar to those of lactate (fig. 3), the most striking difference being seen in blood-samples taken after 30 minutes' exercise.

Glucose.—Changes in blood-glucose level were less striking (fig. 4): resting values were lower in athletes than in non-athletes; at the end of 30 minutes of exercise the values for the athletes were above resting levels, whereas the untrained subjects had the same or slightly lower values.

Glycerol.—Blood-levels were slightly lower in the athletes at rest than in the non-athletes, and in both groups the concentration rose to similar values during exercise and then declined after exercise (fig. 5).

F.F.A.—Plasma-F.F.A. levels at the start of the experiment were lower in the trained subjects compared with the untrained group, but this was not significant ($p \geqslant 0.05$). After 30 minutes of running, the mean F.F.A. levels were 0·45 and 0·65 µeq. per ml., respectively. At the end of the exercise period, the concentrations were greatly elevated in the untrained subjects, whereas there was a much smaller increase in the values for athletes (fig. 6). This difference between the two groups was maintained in the post-exercise period.

Ketone bodies.—Blood ketone-body concentrations (acetoacetate plus 3-hydroxybutyrate) also rose during and after exercise. The athletes, however, showed only a slight rise throughout the experimental period, while in the untrained subjects they rose strikingly in the post-exercise period (fig. 7). The mean hydroxybutyrate/acetoacetate ratios were similar in both groups (range 1·6–2·2) during exercise, but were somewhat higher in the untrained subjects (2·8–3·3) compared with the athletes (2·3–2·7) during the recovery period.

Discussion

The trained and untrained subjects, differing considerably in their running speed and the accompanying physiological characteristics (lower heart-rates and higher weight-losses in the trained subjects), showed clearcut differences in the concentrations of metabolites

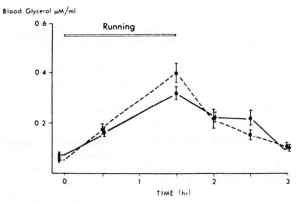

Fig. 5—Changes in blood-glycerol (symbols as in fig. 1).

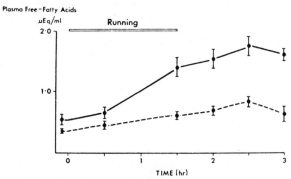

Fig. 6—Changes in plasma-F.F.A. (symbols as in fig. 1).

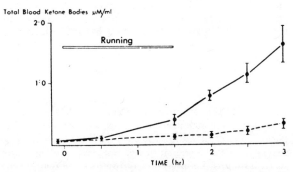

Fig. 7—Changes in blood-ketone-bodies (symbols as in fig. 1).

related to energy supply. The blood-lactate concentration rose by only 0·18 μmole per ml. in the athletes but by 3·49 μmole per ml. in the untrained subjects after 30 minutes of exercise. During the ensuing 60 minutes of running the lactate concentration of the untrained subjects dropped whilst that of the trained subjects rose only slightly. The changes in pyruvate generally paralleled those of lactate in both groups. Lower concentrations of lactate and pyruvate in blood of athletes during exercise have been observed by several workers.[10-13] Thus athletes either produce less lactate during the early stages of exercise or they dispose of it more rapidly. Increased disposal could be due to an increased rate of oxidation in muscle or to an accelerated rate of hepatic gluconeogenesis from lactate.

F.F.A. levels rose steadily in both groups during exercise, but whilst it doubled approximately in the athletes it trebled in the untrained group after $1^1/_2$ hours. This striking difference could be due to either the athletes mobilising less fat or utilising it more quickly. The amount of glycerol appearing in the venous blood may be taken as a guide to changes in adipose-tissue lipolysis, and since the increase in glycerol during exercise was similar in both groups we assume that there was no major difference in fat mobilisation between the athletes and non-athletes. The F.F.A./glycerol ratio was similar in both groups (about 7) before the start of exercise but was considerably lower in the athletes (1·5–2·5) compared with the non-athletes (4) during exercise; this difference was maintained during the recovery period. This suggests that athletes can oxidise fatty acids more effectively than can untrained subjects.

The relatively low concentrations of acetoacetate and 3-hydroxybutyrate in both groups during exercise indicate that ketone bodies are unlikely to be an important fuel in this situation because, in the resting animal at least, the rate of ketone-body utilisation seems to be directly related to their concentration in blood.[14 15] This low concentration of ketone bodies during exercise, in contrast to the post-exercise period, may be important in assuring an ample supply of F.F.A. (and glucose), because in high concentration ketone bodies exert both an antilipolytic and hypoglycæmic effect.[16-18] The absence of an appreciable rise in the ketone-body concentration during the post-exercise period in the trained group can in part be explained by the lower F.F.A. concentration, but may also indicate a facilitation of ketone-body utilisation. The approximate parallelism between the concentrations of F.F.A. and ketone bodies after exercise (figs. 6 and 7) suggests that the availability of F.F.A. is an important factor in the development of post-exercise ketosis.

The only metabolite measured which did not show major differences between the two groups was glucose, and this is probably a reflection of its minor role as fuel in the later stages of the type of exercise undertaken in the present study.

182

To what extent the increased disposal of lactate and F.F.A. in athletes during exercise is due to increases in the activities of rate-limiting enzymes or to other factors remains an open question.

We thank students of Glasgow and Oxford universities and members of the Garscube Harriers and Thames Valley Harriers for acting as subjects. This work was supported by the Royal Society, the Medical Research Council, the Medical Commission for Accident Prevention, the Peel Trust, and the U.S. Public Health Service (grant no. AMO8715). Prof. J. A. Simpson and Prof. J. N. Davidson have provided encouragement, and Dr. J. L. Corbett collaborated in early investigations. R. H. J. is in receipt of the E. G. Fearnsides scholarship of the University of Cambridge, and D. H. W. is a member of the external staff of the Medical Research Council.

Requests for reprints should be addressed to R. H. J., Department of Neurology, Killearn Hospital, Killearn, by Glasgow.

REFERENCES

1. Courtice, F. C., Douglas, C. G. *Proc. R. Soc. B.* 1936, **119**, 381.
2. Cooper, K. E., Johnson, R. H., Pugh, L. G. C. E. Unpublished.
3. Pugh, L. G. C. E., Corbett, J. L., Johnson, R. H. *J. appl. Physiol.* 1967, **23**, 347.
4. Åstrand, P.-O., Hallback, I., Hedman, R., Saltin, B. *ibid.* 1963, **18**, 619.
5. Williamson, D. H., Mellanby, J., Krebs, H. A. *Biochem. J.* 1962, **82**, 90.
6. Hohorst, H. J., Kreutz, F. F., Bücher, T. *Biochem. Zeit.* .1959, **332**, 18.
7. Bergmeyer, H. U., Bernt, E. *in* Methods of Enzymatic Analysis (edited by H. U. Bergmeyer); p. 123. Weinheim, 1963.
8. Kreutz, F. *Klin. Wschr.* 1962, **40**, 362.
9. Itaya, K., Ui, M. *J. Lipid Res.* 1965, **6**, 16.
10. Holmgren, A. *Scand. J. clin. Lab. Invest.* 1956, **8**, suppl. no. 24, p. 1.
11. Holmgren, A., Strom, G. *Acta med. scand.* 1959, **163**, 185.
12. Cobb, L. A., Johnson, W. P. *J. clin. Invest.* 1963, **42**, 800.
13. Juchems, R., Kumper, E. *New Engl. J. Med.* 1968, **278**, 913.
14. Nelson, N., Grayman, I., Mirsky, I. A. *J. biol. Chem.* 1941, **140**, 361.
15. Bates, M. W., Krebs, H. A., Williamson, D. H. *Biochem. J.* 1968, **110**, 655.
16. Björntorp, P., Scherstén, T. *Am. J. Physiol.* 1967, **212**, 683.
17. Balasse, E., Ooms, H. A. *Diabetologia*, 1968, **4**, 133.
18. Senior, B., Loridan, L. *Nature, Lond.* 1968, **219**, 83.

HEAT ADAPTATION AND INJURY IN FOOTBALL PLAYERS

HERMAN C. MAGANZINI, M.D., F.A.C.P.

Although deaths among high school and college football players in this country are rare, a few do occur each year. Most of these are accidental and basically not preventible (assuming the usual precautions of adequate equipment, training, etc.). Unfortunately, some of the deaths are due to heat stroke, and these must be considered preventible. From 1960 to 1963 thirty deaths among high school football players were reported and of these five 16% were attributed to heat stroke[1] and therefore presumably preventible. For the 1966 season one of 26 high school football fatalities was due to heat stroke[2]. Certainly many of the late summer and early fall practices and games, in most areas of Maryland are carried on in conditions of temperature and humidity which could be dangerous for the unprepared athlete.

It is the purpose of this paper to present the physiologic problem and hopefully to suggest cer-

Presented at Seminar on the Medical Aspects of Sports, August 14, 1967.

tain prophylactic measures so that no such preventible tragedies occur in the State of Maryland.

PHYSIOLOGY

Heat Production: Of all the energy expended during strenuous physical exercise, approximately 25% generates productive work. The other 75% raises the body temperature. This can cause the central body (core) temperature to be elevated 4 F or more (rectal temperature of 104+F) unless this heat can be properly dissipated.

Heat Dissipation: Heat is lost from the body by one or more of the following four methods: *Radiation*, the loss of heat to objects of surrounding air which is cooler than the body, accounts for approximately 50% of the loss. *Convection*, which requires some air movement, accounts for about 15%. *Evaporation* from the skin and lungs under normal circumstances, accounts for approximately 30%. *Warming* of the inspired air and heating of food and water intake, accounts for the last 5%. Obviously all of these methods of heat loss, except for evaporation, assume that the environment is cooler than the body. Also implied is the absence of insulating clothing and the presence of convection currents of air. The percentage losses outlined are approximated only if the ambient temperature is below 80 F. Above this, evaporation plays an increasingly important role, until at an air temperature of approximately 95 F all modalities, except evaporation of sweat, cease to be significant. This must now account for 100% of any heat loss. In addition to the importance of air temperature, it becomes obvious that the rate of sweat evaporation is inversely proportional to the environmental humidity. The higher the humidity the less evaporation can take place and therefore the less heat can be dissipated by this means. Likewise it can be seen that the amount and type of clothing will influence not only the amount of work necessary to accomplish a given task but also the amount of evaporation which will be allowed.

ACCLIMATIZATION TO HEAT

It has been demonstrated repeatedly that individuals can be trained to better tolerate strenuous exertion in a hot and humid environment. Much of this investigation has been done in the gold mines of South Africa[5] where wet bulb temperatures of 80 F or more constitute the normal working environment. Similar work has also been done by the military in this country[6] and all results are in agreement. This training in the heat causes increased circulation to the skin and dilatation of the skin blood vessels followed by an increase in the blood volume, primarily the extracellular fluid. There is also an increased ability to sweat and to produce larger volumes of dilute sweat for a given amount of work. The same degree of exertion produces less of a rise in body temperature and pulse rate compared to the unacclimatized individual.

These changes allow the person to perform stenuous tasks in high environmental temperature and humidity, without suffering the heat injury which would occur were he not so acclimatized. It has been shown that this adaptation requires that exercise be carried on in the heat. This can be of short duration, perhaps as short as one hour a day, but cannot consist only of exposure to or rest in the heat. This alone will not allow acclimatization to take place and strenuous physical exertion must in fact be carried out in the hot environment. It implies additionally, adequate salt and water intake to replace the losses incurred by sweating as well as to allow expansion of the extracellular fluid volume.

By this method acclimatization to heat begins after several days and is approximately 80% complete in five to seven days. After two weeks of training it is virtually complete.[3,5] It should be noted however that this acclimatization can be lost. In fact approximately 50% is lost after one week with almost none remaining after two weeks.[7] This means that an individual not exercising in the heat for two weeks would require

186

complete retraining prior to taking part again without heat illness.

Obesity and Conditioning: The state of conditioning and training of the individual seems to play a part in the ease with which he adapts to severe exercise in the heat. Piwonka and his associates at Indiana University[8] tested distance runners in April, 1963 who had not been exposed to heat since the previous summer and who should have lost any previous heat acclimatization. The authors postulated that the daily strenuous exertion of running caused frequent changes in the central body temperature with involvement of the temperature regulating responses of sweating and cutaneous blood flow which "preacclimatized" the runners. They could however be acclimatized to a higher degree and were so, beyond that which others not so physically trained, could reach.[9]

It has been observed that obese individuals acclimatize poorly to heat and may have difficulty in becoming acclimatized at all.

THE FOOTBALL PLAYER'S PROBLEM

Many if not most areas of Maryland have the conditions of heat and humidity during late August and September which could cause and have caused heat illness, injury and death among football players. These athletes are susceptible to heat injury for this sport requires extreme exertion. The uniform which they wear has been shown to increase the work load for a given task 70% above that of the same task, performed by the same individual, in a light cloth "scrub" suit.[4] When fully dressed with helmet, shoulder pads and other equipment there is little area exposed for the essential evaporation of sweat.

Many of the boys are overweight and may not be in condition at the end of summer. In this regard it should be noted that of the nine deaths from heat stroke reported in American football from 1956 to 1963 all of the players were considered large for their age and all were interior linemen.[4] Again, demonstrating the fact that some football players may not be in condition and certainly not heat acclimatized at the beginning of football practice, it was noted that of these same deaths five occurred on the first day and two on the second day of fall practice.

THE PREVENTION OF HEAT INJURY

Conditioning: All proposed football candidates should be encouraged by their coaches to start individual training two to four weeks prior to the first organized practice session. This can probably best be done by running. It has been suggested that these boys start with running 220 followed by 440, 880 and three-quarter of a mile and finally be able to run one mile in the heat prior to the first practice. This might accomplish the preacclimatization of training and if performed faithfully in the hot weather, true heat acclimatization as well.

Salt and Water: Once the practice sessions have in fact started, the candidates must be allowed free access to water on both the practice and game field. Frequent breaks must be provided to allow water to be taken in amounts of at least four to six ounces per hour but more may be necessary. This can be given as ice water or as a salt solution of approximately 0.1%. The addition of lemon juice seems to mask the salt taste. Some of these lemon-salt solutions are commercially available but such a solution can be prepared by dissolving one teaspoonful of salt in six quarts of water and adding lemons to taste. Alternately, four teaspoonfuls of salt and six lemons can be added to one bucket of ice water.[10] They must be encouraged to take at least six to 12 salt tablets per day especially during the weeks of acclimatization, in addition to the heavy salting of food. These tablets need not be taken on the practice field but considering the frequent reluctance, it would be worthwhile to see that several are taken before and after practice to insure the intake of at least this amount. It is most important to increase and replace the salt stores of the body on a day to day basis by all available means.

There has been some evidence presented that

188

over-hydration, before exertion in the heat, may be beneficial in preventing the heat problems.[11] It would perhaps be wise to allow free access to water while suiting up and in fact encourage the taking of six to 12 ounces of fluid during this time.

Clothing: Light weight uniforms must be used during this time of the year. They should consist of short sleeved, light weight, loose fitting jerseys without football stockings. Even less clothing than this (see Tables 1 and 2) should be used if the conditions of temperature and humidity dictate. Under no circumstances should rubber suits be allowed. They have no place in weight loss or conditioning and can only cause an excessive loss of fluid with rise in body temperature. Both predispose to heat injury and one death has been reported with the use of a rubber suit, on a day when the wet bulb temperature was only 64 F.[4] Shirts should be changed when soaked during practice and if possible, dry jerseys should be available on game days to be changed at half-time in this type of hot weather. The wet shirt close to the body forms a blanket which allows none of the essential evaporation and again predisposes to heat injury.

An important preventive measure, which should be adopted if at all possible, is the daily weighing of all candidates before and after practice. The serious heat syndromes are caused primarily by severe dehydration. This excessive loss of fluid can be appreciated prior to the occurrence of any symptoms by careful weighing. The average weight loss in a conditioned athlete will be about five pounds per practice, most of which will be regained by the next day. Any boy approaching a ten pound weight loss must be observed very carefully for this represents a fluid loss of approximately five liters. It must be insisted that he increase his intake of water on the field as well as his intake of salt tablets at home and during the day. He must be observed for the early signs of heat exhaustion. As heat acclimatization is reached, the daily weight loss will decrease as well, and therefore it can serve as an index of adaptation. As previously mentioned, the overweight or poorly conditioned individual must be watched more closely than others and these boys especially should be weighed carefully before and after practice.

Practice Schedule: On days of extreme heat and humidity practices could be held before 10 am or after 6 pm, the coolest parts of the day. The temperature and humidity should be determined daily prior to the start of each session and most logically it would be best to measure them on the actual playing field. This is best done with a "sling psychrometer" which is relatively inexpensive and which measures both temperature and relative humidity. If this is not feasible then a telephone call to the nearest airport or weather station would give the general local conditions and might be sufficient. Suggested practice schedules and clothing are listed in Tables 1 and 2. The wet bulb temperatures of Table 2 can be directly determined from the psychrometer.

Stimulants: and certain weight reducing drugs have been responsible for deaths in athletes and should be forbidden.[1]

HEAT ILLNESS AND INJURY

A clue to the athlete suffering heat illness is the loss of mental accuracy and alertness as well as the onset of awkwardness and lethargy. Fatigue caused by strenuous exertion is manifested by a decrease in activity whereas heat symptoms are those of poor intellectual performance.

Heat Cramps: Muscular cramps most commonly in the calves of the legs (gastrocnemius) are minor symptoms. These are usually due to inadequate salt intake and seem to be worse during games rather than practice, perhaps because of the excessive sweating sustained under emotional stress. The best treatment is prevention by means

TABLE 1
SUGGESTED PRACTICE SCHEDULE*

Temperature	Humidity	Activities
Less than 80 F.		No restrictions.
80 to 90 F	Less than 70%	Watch carefully.
80 to 90 F	More than 70%	Ten minutes rest each hr. Change
90 to 100 F	Less than 70%	T - shirts when wet Observe carefully
90 to 100 F	More than 70%	Discontinue prac-
More than 100 F	Regardless	tice or very short program in shorts and T-shirts

*Modified from Murphy, R. J. (1)

of adequate salt and water intake as well as acclimatization. When they do occur, firm pressure over the area of the cramp will usually relieve the spasm. Some dilute salt solution should be administered. The athlete may return to play but should be watched for the onset of more serious heat symptoms.

Heat Exhaustion: This is characterized by weakness, fatigue, faintness, and excessive perspiration with a cool skin. The breathing becomes rapid but the body temperature is usually normal or only slightly elevated. Nausea, vomiting and restlessness may occur. This is a more serious sign of heat injury and should be treated by the removal of as much clothing and equipment as possible. The athlete should be placed at rest and cooled rapidly with fans or ice packs and dilute salt water administered. He should also be watched carefully for decreasing perspiration and increasing body temperature. This athlete should not be allowed to play further.

TABLE 2
SUGGESTED PRACTICE SCHEDULE
(WET BULB TEMP.)*

Temperature (wet bulb)	Activities
Less than 60 F	No precaution necessary.
61 to 65 F	Alert observation especially the considerable weight losers.
66 to 70 F	Adequate salt and water intake on the field and alert observation.
71 to 75 F	Rest period every thirty minutes in addition to the above.
76 F and higher	Postpone practice or shorts and light T-shirt workout only.

*From Murphy, R. J. and Ashe, W. F. (4)

Heat Stroke: This is a *life threatening emergency* and must be dealt with promptly. In addition to the weakness and faintness there is headache, confusion and ultimately coma. The skin is hot and dry with the absence of sweat and the body temperature rises rapidly. Primary treatment is the rapid lowering of body temperature by removal of clothing and equipment, ice tubs, cold clothes, fans, etc. Immediate hospitalization is essential to avoid permanent damage or death.

SUMMARY

The time available for adequate preparation prior to the start of the football schedule is relatively short. This places great pressures on coaches and players alike to proceed with vigorous, daily training regardless of weather conditions. Heat injury, however, is preventible and the precautions outlined will allow maximum preparation with little loss of practice time, minimum loss of players from heat disability and above all no loss of life from heat stroke. These precautions are:

CONDITIONING: Encourage the athletes to train in the heat prior to the start of regular practice sessions.

WATER: There must be free access to water before and during practices and games, ie. actually present on the field.

SALT: Insist on adequate intake of at least six to twelve tablets per day and more for the heavy weight losers.

TEMPERATURE AND HUMIDITY: Check it daily prior to practice and schedule the gear, type and hour of practice accordingly.

WEIGHT LOSS: Check it for each session with special attention to the losers of ten pounds or more.

OTHER: No stimulants or rubber suits allowed.

HEAT ILLNESS: Know the symptoms and emergency treatment being especially aware of loss of alertness and accuracy.

BIBLIOGRAPHY

1. Murphy, Robert J.: The Problem of Environmental Heat in Athletics. *Ohio State Medical Journal* 59 8:799-804, August 1963.

2. The Twenty-First Annual Report of High School Football Fatalities, 1944-1966. January 1967. Prepared by the National Federation of State High School Athletic Associations.

3 Bass, D. E., Kleeman, C. R., Quinn, M., Henschel, A., and Hegnauer, A. H.: Mechanisms of Acclimatization to Heat in Man. *Medicine* 34:323-380, September 1955.

4. Murphy, Robert J., and Ashe, William F.: Prevention of Heat Illness in Football Players. *JAMA* 194 6:650-654, 8 November 1965.

5. Wyndham, C. H.: Effect of Acclimatization on the Sweat Rate/Rectal Temperature Relationship. *J. Appl. Physiol.* 22 1:27-30, 1967.

6. Stonehill, R. B., and Keil, P. G.: Successful Preventive Measures Against Heal Illness at Lackland Air Force Base. *Amer. J. Public Health* 51:586-590, April 1961.

7. Williams, C. G., Wyndham, C. H., and Morrison, J. F.: Rate of Loss of Acclimatization in Summer and Winter. *J. Appl. Physiol.* 22 1:21-26, January 1967.

8. Piwonka, R. W., Robinson, S., Gay, V. L., and Manalis, R. S.: Preacclimatization of Men to Heat by Training. *J. Appl. Physiol.* 20 3:379-384, 1965.

9. Piwonka, R. W., and Robinson, S.: Acclimatization of Highly Trained Men to Work in Severe Heat. *J. Appl. Physiol.* 22 1:9-12, January 1967.

10. Trickett, Paul C.: Prevention and Treatment of Athletic Injuries. Appleton-Century-Crofts Publications, 1965.

11. Moroff, S. V., and Bass, D. C.: Effects of Over Hydration on Man's Physiological Responses to Work in the Heat. *J. Appl. Physiol.* 20 2:267-270, January 1965.

Alteration of Eccrine Sweat Gland in Fatal Heat Stroke

Electron Microscopic Observation

Nobuhisa Baba, MD, PhD, and Richard D. Ruppert, MD

Light and electron microscopic observations were performed on a biopsy specimen of an eccrine sweat gland obtained from a patient suffering heat stroke. There was marked cellular dehydration, particularly of the basal cells, which are generally considered to secrete water and electrolytes. Such morphological change is believed to reflect the severe fatigue of sweat glands often reported in individuals with heat stroke.

THE MOST adverse effect of heat dissipation is heat stroke, in which hyperpyrexia, central nervous system dysfunctions, and circulatory failure are often followed by fatal outcome. Heat stroke is more often seen in such excessively high environmental temperature and high relative humidity that heat dissipation depends solely upon perspiration. In their classical review of 125 fatal cases of heat stroke, Malamud et al described 88 patients having some disturbances of perspiration.[1] Ferris et al noted absence of sweating in all of the patients with heat stroke as observed by them at the time of admission.[2] It is well known that those patients with congenital absence of sweat glands are extremely sensitive to heat.[3] Also, anticholinergic drugs can predispose some patients to danger of heat stroke by reducing effective perspiration.[4,5] Schwartz and Itoh noted marked and prolonged decrease in response of sweat glands to intracutaneous injection of methacholine (Mecholyl) chloride in patients with heat stroke.[6] In experimental exposure of human subjects to excessive moist heat, an initial phase of excessive sweating was followed by sudden reduction of sweat, and cessation of sweating preceded or often coincided with syncope.[7,8] This paper is to report ultrastructural alteration of an eccrine sweat gland in a fatal case of heat stroke.

Report of a Case

A high-school student had been practicing football in full uniform for approximately two hours on a hot August day until he suddenly collapsed. History indicated that he had been in excellent health, although he had a previous episode of mild heat prostration in the preceding week. When admitted to a local hospital, his rectal temperature was 42.8 C (109 F) and systolic blood pressure was 90 mm Hg. He was immediately cooled and referred to the Ohio State University Hospital. On admission his temperature was down to 37.8 C (100 F) but his blood pressure was 65/0 mm Hg. He was comatose and showed only slight movement of the extremities. The skin was cyanotic. No sweating was noted, although the skin felt warm. Laboratory data included leukocytosis of 21,400 and decreased platelets; hemoglobin, 17.6 gm/100 cc; serum glutamic oxaloacetic transaminase, 850 units; lactic dehydrogenase, 5,500 units; carbon dioxide combining power, 11 mEq/liter; and arterial blood pH, 7.19. Prothrombin time was prolonged to 49.8 seconds (control 13.8 seconds). Other pertinent biochemical data have been previously reported.[9] Plasma fibrinogen was unmeasurably low, and abnormal fibrinolysin was suspected. In view of the severe metabolic acidosis the patient received sodium bicarbonate and tromethamine (tris-buffer) in addition to fresh blood transfusion and chlorpromazine. However, metabolic acidosis was never corrected; he remained comatose and circulatory collapse continued. He died two days after the onset of heat stroke.

At autopsy the most severely affected parenchymal organs were the liver and kidneys. The liver showed severe fatty and hyaline granular degenerations. There was bilateral cortical necrosis of the kidneys and severe damage to the tubules in the medulla. The pancreas and heart showed foci of hemorrhages and degeneration of parenchymal cells. Of note was the presence of multiple hyaline thrombi in the small arteries and arterioles of the kidneys and in the small

veins and sinusoids of the adrenals. There was extensive neuronal degeneration of the cerebral and cerebellar cortices.

Biopsy Findings in the Eccrine Sweat Gland.— A biopsy of the skin of the lower leg was obtained 14 hours before the patient's death. The specimen was immediately placed in cold 6% buffered glutaraldehyde solution and transferred to cold 1% buffered osmium tetroxide solution. The tissue was then embedded in epoxy phenolic polyurethane resin mixture[10] after ethanol dehydration and propylene oxide infiltration. The plastic blocks were examined for sweat glands by 1μ-thick sections.

In the basal layers of the gland there were extremely dark-stained cells with irregular cell borders, whereas most of the cells lining the lumen stained more lightly, with clear apical vesicles (Fig 1 and 2). In the electron microscope these dark cells also presented markedly increased electron density (Fig 3 and 4). The interdigitations between opposing cells were extremely accentuated. Between such cells intercellular canaliculi were noted often. Such dark appearance of the cells suggested shrinkage due to severe cellular dehydration. The profiles of

Fig 1.—Low-power view of sweat gland shows many dark-stained basal cells (B) away from the lumen (L) (epoxy phenolic polyurethane resin-embedded section, toluidine blue-pyronine stain, × 320).

Fig 2.—High-power view of sweat gland shows dark-stained basal cells (B) and pale-stained tall superficial cells (S) with many apical vesicles (V) (epoxy phenolic polyurethane resin-embedded section, toluidine blue-pyronine stain, × 2,000).

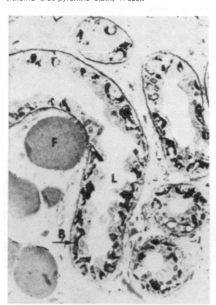

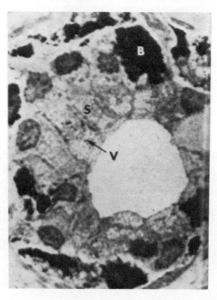

mitochondria were noted in these cells, but other cytoplasmic organelles were not clearly recognized. The areas where glycogen granules had disappeared were electron-pale in contrast to the rest of the darkly-stained cytoplasm. However, these changes were not seen in all of the basal cells, and some basal cells appeared relatively unaffected, even retaining abundant glycogen granules (Fig 5). Most of the superficial cells seemed less changed and showed many

Fig 3.—Basal portion of eccrine sweat gland affected by degeneration. Basal cells (B) surrounding intercellular canaliculus (C) are all electron-dense, indicating severe cellular dehydration. Adjacent myoepithelial cell (M) and superficial cells (S) are less affected by degeneration, and cytoplasmic organelles are recognizable. V is a vesicle in the superficial cell (osmium tetroxide, × 4,300).

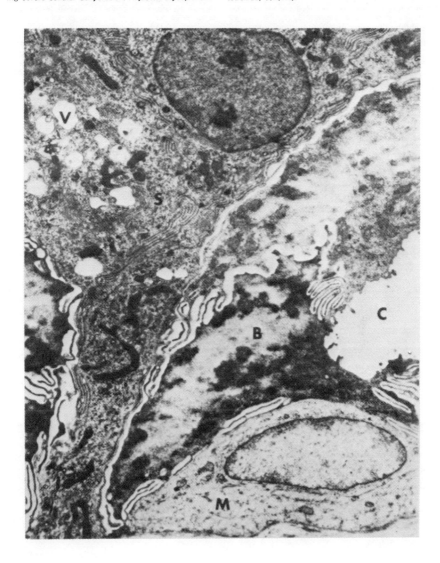

membrane-surrounded clear vesicles near the lumen. In some cells these vesicles contained myelin-like figures. Well-developed Golgi apparatus were noted near the nuclei. Several lipid particles were present. The myoepithelial cells and the endothelial cells of the adjacent capillaries seemed free of degenerative process.

Comment

The terminal coil of the human eccrine sweat gland consists of superficial and basal epithelial cells and myoepithelial cells.[11] In the histological preparations stained with basic dyes, the superficial

Fig 4.—Basal portion of eccrine sweat gland affected by degeneration. Basal cell (B) is extremely electron-dense, indicating cellular dehydration. Except for lipid droplet (L), cytoplasmic organelles are hardly recognizable. Superficial cells (S) are tall and show many cytoplasmic organelles. Numerous vesicles (V) are seen in apical portion of superficial cells (osmium tetroxide. × 6,400).

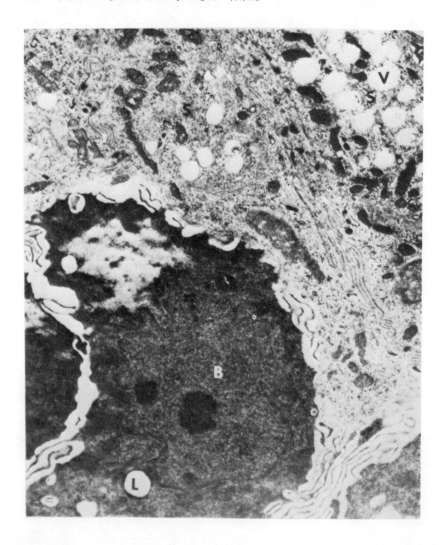

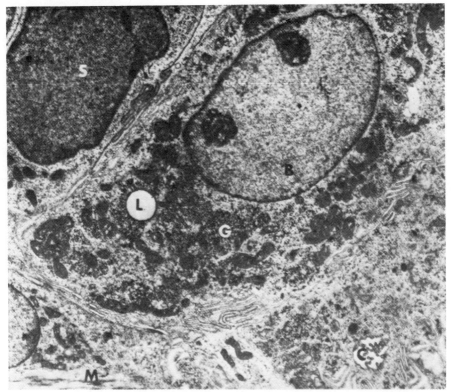

Fig 5.—Basal portion of eccrine sweat gland unaffected by degeneration, showing normal structure. Basal cells (B) show abundant glycogen granules (G). Lipid droplet (L) and small opening of intercellular canaliculus (C) are seen. Myoepithelial cells (M) are located immediately upon basement membrane. Superficial cells (S) contain little glycogen (osmium tetroxide, × 6,400).

cells are dark, and the basal cells are pale. The basal cells are located on the basement membrane or on the myoepithelial cells, and often surround intercellular canaliculi. The superficial cells contain acid mucopolysaccharides and the basal cells are rich in glycogen.[12] The electron microscopic view of such cells has been documented by several investigators.[13-17] The superficial cells show membrane-bound secretory vesicles, whereas the basal cells show no secretory vesicles and less developed endoplasmic reticulum and Golgi apparatus than the former cell type. It has been postulated that the superficial cells are engaged in production of aqueous and electrolyte components of sweat.[15]

At light microscopy level, Dobson et al showed that after profuse sweating, the glycogen contents of the secretory coil and duct were depleted and the superficial cells lost their granules.[18] After daily repetition of profuse sweating, a major change was seen, mainly in the basal cells. It consisted of degeneration (shrinkage, vacuolation and fusion) of these cells.[19] Such effect was markedly enhanced in salt-depleted individuals, in whom progressive atrophy of basal cells was noted.[20] Our finding of severe ultrastructural alterations of the eccrine sweat gland corresponds to the fatigue of the gland as shown in these experiments at the level of light microscopy. It is of note that these changes were more prominent in the basal cells, which are generally considered to secrete water and electrolytes, thus playing a major role in heat dissipation.

Generic and Trade Names of Drugs

Methacholine chloride—*Mecholyl.*
Tromethamine—*Trizma, Tris Amino.*
Chlorpromazine—*Thorazine.*

References

1. Malamud, N.; Haymaker, W.; and Chester, R.P.: Heat Stroke: A Clinicopathologic Study of 125 Cases, *Milit Surgeon,* 99:297-449, 1946.
2. Ferris, E.B., Jr., et al: Heat Stroke: Clinical and Chemical Observations on 44 Cases, *J Clin Invest* 17:249-262, 1938.
3. MacQuaide, D.H.G.: Congenital Absence of Sweat Glands, *Lancet* 2:531-532, 1944.
4. Litman, R.E.: Heat Sensitivity to Autonomic Drugs, *JAMA* 149:635-636 (June 14) 1952.
5. Befeler, D.: Heat Illness With Anhydrosis, *Amer J Gastroent* 44:149-151, 1962.
6. Schwartz, I.L., and Itoh, S.: Fatigue of the Sweat Glands in Heat Stroke, *J Clin Invest* 35: 733-734, 1956.
7. Kuo, K.W., et al, cited by Kuno, Y.: *Human Perspiration,* Springfield, Ill: Charles C Thomas, Publisher, 1956, pp 184-188.
8. Lee, S.T.: Observations on Men Exposed to Excessive Humid Heat, *Jap J Physiol* 2:103-110, 1951.
9. Ruppert, R.D., et al: The Mechanisms of Metabolic Acidosis in Heat Stroke, *Clin Res* 12: 356, 1964.
10. Spurlock, B.D.; Kattine, V.C.; and Freeman, J.A.: A New Epoxy Embedment for Electron Microscopy, *J Cell Biol* 17:203-207, 1962.
11. Ito, T., and Iwashige, K.: Zytologische Untersuchugen über die ekkrine Schweissdrusen in menschlichen Achselhaut mit besonderer Berück-

sichtungen der apokrinen Sekretion derselben. *Okajima Folia Anat Jap* 23:147-165, 1951.
12. Montagna, W.: *The Structure and Function of Skin.* ed 2, New York: Academic Press, 1962. p 454.
13. Hibbs, R.G.: The Fine Structure of Human Eccrine Sweat Glands, *Amer J Anat* 103:201-207, 1958.
14. Charles, A.: An Electron Microscope Study of the Eccrine Sweat Gland, *J Invest Derm* 34:81-88, 1960.
15. Munger, B.L.: The Ultrastructure and Histopathology of Human Eccrine Sweat Glands, *J Biophys Biochem Cytol* 11:385-402, 1961.
16. Ellis, R.A.: The Fine Structure of the Eccrine Sweat Gland, *Advances Biol Skin* 3:30-53, 1962.
17. Zelickson, A.S.: *Electron Microscopy of Skin and Mucous Membrane,* Springfield, Ill: Charles C Thomas, Publisher, 1963.
18. Dobson, R.L., et al: Some Histochemical Observations on Human Eccrine Sweat Glands: III The Effect of Profuse Sweating, *J Invest Derm* 31:147-159, 1958.
19. Dobson, R.L.: The Effect of Repeated Episodes of Profuse Sweating of the Human Eccrine Sweat Glands, *J Invest Derm* 35:195-198, 1960.
20. Dobson, R.L.; Abele, D.C.; and Hale, D.M.: The Effects of High and Low Salt Intake and Repeated Episodes of Sweating on the Human Eccrine Sweat Glands, *J Invest Derm* 36:327-335, 1961.

AUTHOR INDEX

KEY-WORD TITLE INDEX